W9-BRX-581

Also by NICHOLAS PERRICONE, M.D.

The Wrinkle Cure

The Perricone Prescription

The Perricone Prescription Personal Journal

The Acne Prescription

The Clear Skin Prescription

The Perricone Promise

The Perricone Weight-Loss Diet

The Perricone Weight-Loss Diet Personal Daily Journal

Dr. Perricone's 7 Secrets to Beauty, Health, and Longevity

Ageless Face,
Ageless Mind

BALLANTINE BOOKS

NEW YORK

Nicholas Perricone, M.D.

Ageless Face, Ageless Mind

Erase Wrinkles and
Rejuvenate the Brain

Copyright © 2007 by Nicholas V. Perricone, M.D.

Published in the United States by Ballantine Books,
an imprint of The Random House Publishing Group,
a division of Random House, Inc., New York.

BALLANTINE and colophon are registered
trademarks of Random House, Inc.

LIBRARY OF CONGRESS CATALOGING-IN-PUBLICATION DATA
Perricone, Nicholas.
Ageless face, ageless mind : erase wrinkles and
rejuvenate the brain / Nicholas Perricone.
p. cm.
Includes bibliographical references and index.
ISBN 978-0-345-49936-3 (hardcover : alk. paper)
1. Longevity.   2. Glycation.   3. Glycoconjugates—Toxicology.   I. Title.
RA776.75.P474 2008
613'.04244—dc22   2007030558

Printed in the United States of America on acid-free paper

www.ballantinebooks.com

2 4 6 8 9 7 5 3 1

FIRST EDITION

Book design by Jessica Shatan Heslin/Studio Shatan, Inc.

Acknowledgments

Anne Sellaro again deserves star billing in these acknowledgments. Anne's untiring enthusiasm, hard work, creativity, and vision as friend, agent, producer, and collaborator continue to help me share my message and mission with millions of people worldwide.

I would like to extend a warm thank you to the great many friends and colleagues who have generously assisted me including Caroline Sutton, Gina Centrello, Libby McGuire, Tom Perry, Kim Hovey, Brian McLendon, Rachel Bernstein, Cindy Murray, Lisa Barnes, Christina Duffy, and the entire team at Ballantine including their outstanding sales force.

To my many friends and colleagues for their ongoing dedication and support:

David Vigliano and the team at Vigliano Associates
Tony Tiano, Lennlee Keep, Eli Brown and team at Santa Fe Productions
The Public Broadcasting Service (PBS-TV)
Harry G. Preuss, M.D., M.A.C.N., C.N.S.
Michigan State University College of Human Medicine
Department of Dermatology Henry Ford Hospital
The team at the NV Perricone M.D. Flagship Store
The team at NV Perricone M.D. Ltd.
Ken Starr
Johnna Schlosser
Maria La Rosa
Dana Bledsoe

Edward Magnotti

Craig Weatherby

Sharyn Kolberg

Chim Potini

Mahnaz Badamchian

Terence Sellaro

Randy Hartnell and the team at Vital Choice

Our retail partners Sephora, Nordstom, Neiman Marcus,
Bloomingdale's, Saks Fifth Avenue, Henri Bendel, Belk & Parisian

Bob Terry, Ph.D. and Judy Brown at Green Foods

Amy Weitz at InterHealth Nutraceuticals, Inc.

My parents

My children, daughter Caitie, sons Jeffrey, Nicholas, daughter-in-law
Paige, and grandson Nicholas Perricone III

My brother and sisters, Jimmy, Laura, Barbara, and June

Contents

Introduction

A decade ago, when my first book, *The Wrinkle Cure*, appeared, it was considered revolutionary because it revealed the connection between inflammation and aging. However, as time passed the book accomplished its mission, as the role of inflammation in aging and disease became recognized and accepted by the mainstream scientific community. Since then I have explored many other groundbreaking discoveries, including the miracle of cellular rejuvenation, which shows us that we can rebuild our bodies by beginning at the cellular level.

However, in *Ageless Face, Ageless Mind*, I take a giant step into the future. For the first time, I explain one of the cardinal processes of aging. I examine the process that creates Advanced Glycation End Products, appropriately known as AGEs. I introduce the revolutionary and reveal the ultimate in new technology—a technology that will help reverse the effects of AGEs in every organ system, as well as the vast majority of diseases long thought to be part of "normal" aging.

AGEs lie at the very heart of the aging process across all specialties from the skin to the brain. AGEs can be responsible for wrinkles, heart disease, cancer, diabetes, and much more, including age-related memory loss and even Alzheimer's disease. For many years, science has known about AGEs but we have had no effective strategic interventions to fight them—until now. Because of major recent breakthroughs, we can now both control and prevent their deleterious effects. First I target the foods and recipes that will stop and even reverse the formation of AGEs. You will quickly look, feel, and think better as you adopt this way of eating.

Also included is cutting-edge information about supplements that have the power to help you look and feel, well, AGE-less. This includes a technological breakthrough with glutathione, the most powerful, most versatile, and most important of the body's self-generated antioxidants, and some amazing new discoveries about how carnosine can protect your eyes and resveratrol can protect against nearly every age-related disease. You will also be introduced to Pycnogenol®, a unique antioxidant that is vital to health as well as to the collagen and elastin in your skin. These are just a few of the wonderful supplements we now have to help us counter the destructive effects of advanced glycation end products.

But food and supplements are only part of the new strategies to fight AGEs. Rejuvenating the body through skin-derived stem cells is now a viable reality. Initially there was negative publicity connected to stem-cell therapy. This was because stem cells were originally harvested from fetuses, raising many ethical and moral issues that are unresolved to this day.

However, there has been a breakthrough; science has now developed to the point where stem cells can be harvested using a special technique *and* they can be derived from everyone—from infancy through adulthood.

I have had the fortunate opportunity to work side by side with the scientists at the forefront of this new stem-cell technology, researching the potential benefits for my patients and readers throughout the world.

In the following chapters you will learn how this incredible technology can reverse damage from AGEs to rejuvenate skin, and when needed, can be used to combat everything from autoimmune disease to diabetes.

This is science at its most innovative and rewarding, new information that is as fresh, exciting, and advanced as that found in *The Wrinkle Cure* a decade ago.

Join me on this exciting journey as I translate this magic into practical lifestyle applications for total body and mind rejuvenation.

NICHOLAS PERRICONE, M.D.
Madison, CT

PART ONE

The Secret
of the AGEs

Understanding Advanced
Glycation End Products (AGEs)

t is a universal fact that people everywhere desire to look and feel their best, regardless of chronological age.

You would think that teaching people that eating correctly and following a healthy lifestyle would prolong the quality and length of their lives, help prevent degenerative diseases from Alzheimer's to cancer, and fight against vision problems, heart disease, diabetes, obesity, arthritis, and more would be enough to motivate them to take better care of themselves. Unfortunately, in today's world, the message often falls on deaf ears.

Surprisingly, it's often vanity that saves the day. When people hear that they can radically affect the way they *look*, decrease and help prevent deep wrinkles and sagging skin, lose body fat, maintain muscle mass, and increase energy and athletic performance, they become very interested. While often perceived as a shallow trait, vanity is actually one of the greatest of human motivators—and no amount of teaching or preaching about health can quite compare with its transformative powers.

And that's a good thing, because how we look physically is not just about aesthetics or attractiveness. Our skin and outward appearance are accurate reflections of what is going on internally—the state of our internal organs, hormone levels, and overall physiology.

Why is that? What is happening to our outsides that so mirrors our insides?

What's happening is that we are forming AGEs, which—to put it simply—are among the most age-accelerating substances known to science.

WHAT WRINKLES TELL US

Some wrinkles tell us that we've had a hard life. Some tell us that we've spent too much time in the sun. Some tell us that we're getting older, and some tell us that we've inherited a grandparent's face. But *all* wrinkles tell us that the deep lines and sagging skin we see are partial by-products of a process known as *glycation.* Glycation occurs when a glucose (sugar) molecule binds to a protein molecule without the influence of enzymes, proteins that accelerate the rate of chemical reactions. In scientific terms we refer to these sugar/protein bondings as AGEs, an appropriate acronym for *advanced glycation end products.*

While wrinkled skin is one of the visible appearances of AGEs, most degenerative diseases are affected in one way or another by disease-producing glycation reactions. These reactions result in major damage to the body, including arterial stiffening; atherosclerosis (the clogging, narrowing, and hardening of the blood vessels); the formation of cataracts; neurological impairment; diabetic complications; and wrinkled, sagging skin. In other words, the formation of AGEs is responsible for serious damage to the body, both internally and externally.

BREAKING THROUGH THE AGEs BARRIER

For years, scientists have thought that there was no way to reverse the effects of AGEs. They have tried to develop anti-glycating drugs, all of which have been proven to be either ineffectual or potentially dangerous.

That is why this book is so important. For the first time, you will read about breakthrough strategies to stop and prevent the damage AGEs can cause. *Ageless Face, Ageless Mind* teaches you how to holistically reverse the visible damage to skin in the form of wrinkles, sagging, and loss of tone and contour, as well as the invisible, internal damage in all organ systems, including age-related memory loss. You will learn:

- How AGEs are formed inside the body, resulting in serious damage to skin and all organ systems;

- How AGEs are as widespread and detrimental in processed food as trans fats and high-fructose corn syrup;

- How it's not only the foods you eat, but the way they're prepared that influences the glycation process. You will also learn the best cooking methods to avoid their formation;

- How to offset the AGEing mechanism with safe, effective, targeted nutritional supplements that will prevent the glycation reaction—at the exact moment that the glycation is occurring—for example, when you eat sweets or grilled meats; and

- How AGEs help create and exacerbate the deleterious effects of inflammation—now familiar to all Perricone readers—and perhaps most important, how you can control it and reverse many of its negative consequences.

In this book, I introduce you to a supplement that can save your eyesight, and a potent drink that can detoxify your system, even when you've had too much alcohol. You'll learn what to eat (and more important, what to avoid eating), and how important certain types of exercises can be to stave off the AGEing process. And you'll discover how groundbreaking stem cell science has been used to develop topical formulas that keep AGEs from making you look older than you really are.

Although my initial focus is always on creating and maintaining youthful, beautiful, and healthy skin, by controlling and even reversing AGEs we can now reap huge additional benefits. We can

- Prevent insulin resistance, the precursor to Metabolic Syndrome

- Prevent diabetes and help alleviate symptoms in diabetes sufferers

- Control the processes leading to Alzheimer's disease

- Prevent vascular disease

- Protect the retina and preserve eyesight

- Prevent kidney disease and impaired kidney function

- Prevent cataracts

- Prevent loss of memory and diminished brain power (neurodegeneration)

- Prevent cardiovascular disease

- Prevent the chromosomal instability that leads to cancer

After decades of research we are finally getting closer to solving the mystery of how to safely and effectively prevent AGEs' deadly and disfiguring effects.

AGES ACCELERATE AGING

Western medicine is divided into hundreds of different specialties. The neurologist studies and treats the brain; the dermatologist's focus is the skin, hair, and nails; the ophthalmologist's the eyes; the gerontologist's aging; the cardiologist's the heart; and so forth. However, AGEs cut across the myriad medical specialties, and its study compels us to create treatments that are truly holistic. While there is not one definitive cause of aging, the different pathways—including inflammation, insulin imbalance, and AGEs—are closely interconnected. All three are major players in the physical and mental deterioration that often accompany aging, accelerating with each decade.

The reason for this is the simple fact that our bodies are composed mainly of protein, and protein is responsible for the daily functioning of the body. AGEs are highly destructive to this protein. When the integrity of the body's protein is threatened or compromised, there is a significant impact on both the body's function and appearance.

As we age, the protein in our bodies begins to deteriorate. This is due in large part to the damaging effects of aldehydes, which are a class of highly reactive chemical compounds and sugar. Aldehydes do their damage by accumulating in the body from such diverse sources as alcohol intake, cigarette smoking, vehicle exhaust fumes, and even chronic Candida infections.

Aldehydes also decrease energy production by inhibiting coenzyme A, which is present in all living cells and essential to the metabolism of carbohydrates, fats, and some amino acids. Chronic aldehyde exposure also contributes to numerous signs and symptoms of aging, including heart disease and cataracts, and has damaging effects on brain function.

How AGEs Form

It all starts with sugar. All sugar molecules can be linear (think of a straight piece of string on a table) or they can cyclize (that is, form a circle by connecting both ends). At normal body pH (acid-alkaline balance) most of our glucose is in a circle. This is the good news, because the circle is more stable. Unfortunately, the remainder of the glucose is in the straight or linear form, which is highly reactive. It is this linear glucose that attaches to our proteins. This attachment is called *cross-linking*, a phrase that comes up over and over again in AGE research. Cross-linking, or glycation, is the result of AGEs. These three terms—cross-linking, glycation, and AGEs—are often used synonymously, because each describes the end result of AGE formation. In other words, the cross-linking or glycating of proteins results in the formation of Advanced Glycation End Products.

To visualize this process in action, imagine that you are building a ladder. Start with the two long side pieces and a box full of short cross pieces, the rungs, which will act as the steps of the ladder. The long side pieces represent proteins. The short rungs represent sugar (glucose).

When we begin, the two long side pieces of the ladder are not connected by any rungs. In other words, the proteins in our body are free flowing, with a lot of space for water between them.

Now we take the two long side pieces of the ladder and add one "rung." The rung (sugar) has just connected or cross-linked the two proteins, making them stiffer and less flexible and free flowing. As the years go by, more and more sugar rungs are added to the protein side pieces, making the proteins more rigid.

As you can imagine, once the ladder has been built by connecting the sugar rungs to the protein side pieces, there is very little space for water inside the ladder compared to when the two long side pieces were not connected. This is what creates the serious problem of altered proteins. Once the structure and function of the proteins have been altered, they can no longer effectively fulfill their critical roles.

Save Your Protein

Protein degradation and malfunction is a major cause of aging, and can be the result of attacks on proteins by other molecules. If glycation gets out of hand, many proteins that are vitally important for the proper functioning of the body will be degraded or destroyed. Our natural ability to protect against glycation declines with age, which in turn leads to increasing glycation damage. A critical enzyme involved in protection against glycation is glyoxalase 1. Using a model system involving the nematode worm, *Caenorhabditis elegans*, which has been studied extensively in the field of life extension, Professor Paul Thornalley of the University of Warwick and his collaborators at the University of Heidelburg have shown for the first time that by enhancing levels of glyoxalase 1 the glycation process can be diminished, and life can be extended by up to 40%! Similarly, by decreasing amounts of the enzyme, they have shortened the life span of the nematodes. I concur with Thornalley's conclusion that *"this implies that glycation promotes multiple types of protein damage in aging."*

Of course, humans are quite a bit different from nematodes. However, any substance that can undo the incalculable damage of AGEs deserves additional research.

AGES INSIDE AND OUT

The first step in prevention is to understand why these AGEs form in the first place and where they come from. AGEs can be exogenous, that is, produced outside the body, or endogenous, produced inside the body.

AGEs from the Inside

As we now know, AGEs form when a sugar molecule attaches to a protein without the controlling action of an enzyme. Scientists call this a nonenzymatic reaction. Proteins are the basic building blocks of life. They are comprised of amino acids, make up much of the body's tissue, and are necessary for the structure, function, and regulation of the body's cells, tissues, and organs. Each protein has its own unique functions. Proteins can act as hormones (some hormones that are products of endocrine glands are proteins or peptides; others are steroids), enzymes, antibodies, structural components, or signaling molecules. Enzymes, for example, are proteins produced by living cells that facilitate specific chemical or metabolic reactions throughout the body. An antibody is a protein produced by the body's immune system that recognizes and helps fight infections and other foreign substances in the body. And collagen is an insoluble, structural protein fiber that is the primary constituent of connective tissue (skin and cartilage), providing support to bones, tendons, and skin.

At the point where sugar attaches to a protein, there is a small mechanism creating inflammation. When these sugar molecules attach to collagen protein, for example, wrinkles are formed as the inflammation produces enzymes that break down the collagen. This process also causes the cross-linking described earlier, making the collagen stiff and inflexible where it was once soft and supple, similar to what happens when you leave a fine kid-leather glove out in the rain.

We produce endogenous AGEs when we take in sugar and foods that rapidly convert to sugar, such as high-glycemic carbohydrates, including potatoes, baked goods, breads, pasta, bagels, and chips. These foods cause sudden spikes in blood sugar levels, resulting in a burst of inflammation and the release of insulin into the bloodstream. This sugar attaches to the proteins in our body, resulting in the formation of AGEs, which are free-radical factories (and free radicals are the primary force behind our old enemy, inflammation).

These "sugar bonds" can occur throughout the body as we age. The sugar molecule attaches itself to collagen, which is found in our arteries, skin, veins, bones, ligaments, and even our brains, resulting in the breakdown of organ systems and the deterioration of the body. AGEs have also been found in other proteins in the body, including the extracellular matrix (any material produced by cells and secreted into the surrounding medium), the brain, the cartilage between joints, the kidneys, and the lens of the eyes, where their accumulation leads to a cross-link with proteins that play a pivotal role in the formation of cataracts.

AGEs slowly build up over time. As we get older this ongoing, destructive process compromises essential proteins in the body. Because the structure and function of the proteins has been altered, they can no longer effectively fulfill their critical roles. To circumvent this process, we need to maintain even levels of blood sugar and insulin. A good way to do this is to avoid sugary and starchy foods and beverages as much as possible. In later chapters you will learn what nutrients and nutritional supplements can help you maintain healthy blood-sugar levels and block the formation of AGEs

AGEs from the Outside

As if producing AGEs inside our bodies wasn't enough, we also consume preformed AGEs through some of the foods we eat. Recent studies have provided evidence that certain foods are significant exogenous sources of highly reactive AGEs. Modern methods of food processing, especially the heating of sugars with proteins or fat, accelerate their formation. Fried and processed foods promote their formation, as does dark roasting—whether of meats, coffee beans, or nuts. Deeply browned baked goods are also implicated. Here's how it works.

When sugar (glucose) reacts with amino acids in proteins, it creates brown-colored cross-linked structures. This process is known as the Maillard (or browning) reaction, first described by Louis Maillard in 1912. Toasting a piece of bread or roasting a turkey to a golden brown produces the Maillard reaction, which darkens and toughens foods. The Maillard reaction is an important part of much food processing. Many of its effects, including the caramel aromas and rich, golden-brown colors, are what makes food so appealing. In recent decades, food manufacturers have used this knowledge to boost the flavor of natural foods by incorporating synthetic AGEs into them. This has resulted in a vast increase in the AGE content of foods over the past 50 years—and these AGEs can be just as damaging as other ingredients we now know to be toxic to our health, including trans fats, chemical preservatives, and high-fructose corn syrup. Even though food manufacturers know that many of these additives and methods of preparation are extremely detrimental to our health, they refuse to take action.

A perfect example is the trans fats fiasco. It is only because of public awareness and outcry that some manufacturers are now removing trans fats from their products. Unfortunately, some the biggest users of trans fats are manufacturers of foods such as cookies and sweet baked goods that are targeted to children. Many fast food chains are now advertising that they have found new ingredients in which to cook their fries and onion rings—although not all have yet begun to use these ingredients. In late 2006, the New York City Board of Health voted to make New York the nation's first city to outlaw the use of artery-clogging artificial trans fats in restaurants. This includes elegant bistros, neighborhood pizzerias, and bakeries both large and small. While these are steps in the right direction, all they've really done is make many foods, such as doughnuts and fries, a little less unhealthy with the trans fat removal. However, they can still promote AGE formation and are still causing our bodies great harm!

Although it provides desirable flavor and aroma, the Maillard reaction also reduces the nutritional properties of food, affecting protein availability by destroying vitamin content and inhibiting digestive enzymes. It also promotes the formation of potentially toxic substances that can cause alterations in cell DNA. These mutagenic compounds, which cause a permanent change in the genetic material in each living cell, can be carcinogenic—another compelling reason to choose foods in their most natural, least-processed state.

When we process potatoes in the form of French fries or potato chips, we are using oil heated to a very high heat. In fact, most junk or popular snack food is prepared using extremely high temperatures, leading to the formation of AGEs and gene-mutating toxins better known as carcinogens. Sugar is also often added to chips, fries, and baked goods to accelerate the browning process, which, unfortunately, also accelerates AGEs.

But it's not only cooking proteins at high heats that creates AGEs. Cooking them at low heats can also create AGEs. Cooking foods for extended periods, such as slow grilling or barbecuing meats or caramelizing onions and other vegetables or fruits in a sauté pan, also leads to the formation of AGEs.

If we shouldn't cook foods at high heat or low heat, what's left? Fortunately, there are things we can do to enjoy delicious, AGE-free foods. For instance, keeping the concept of the "browning" reaction in mind, we can sauté vegetables such as onions to the transparency stage but not brown them to the caramelization stage. And, as you will learn later, by marinating and/or basting most foods prior to or during cooking, we can cut way back on the AGEs created.

The Case Against High Heat

As we have learned, it isn't just charbroiled meats that cause AGE formation. Cooking vegetables at high heat, especially starchy ones like potatoes, can also create a carcinogenic substance known as acrylamide. Acrylamide is a chemical created in foods when starches and other carbohydrates are overheated (over 120° C or 250° F) during cooking. Acrylamide is also used in papermaking, ore processing, permanent-press fabrics, dye manufacture, and wastewater (sewage) treatment.

Although most consumers have not heard of acrylamide, a lot of attention has been given to the issue of acrylamide in foods by both the Food and Drug Administration (FDA) and the World Health Organization (WHO). According to the FDA, scientists around the world are trying to determine exactly how acrylamide is formed in food. Richard Stadler of the Nestle Research Center in Lausanne, Switzerland, and Donald Mottram of Britain's University of Reading reported in the journal *Nature* that they found that the Maillard reaction may explain how acrylamide forms in food. They discovered that the amino acid asparagine has the potential to become an acrylamide during the Maillard reaction. This occurs at temperatures above 100° C (212° F).

Scientists have found that potato chips, particularly the dark russet variety, and French fries have dangerously high levels of acrylamide, and that there is a strong link between acrylamide consumption and the risk of developing cancer. FDA researchers have found that acrylamide damages DNA and cell proteins. Such damage is often a first step to cancer, because it can lead to mutations that cause cells to grow into tumors.

Acrylamide does not appear to be present or is present at nondetectable levels in uncooked foods.

Although it appears that cooking methods such as frying, roasting, grilling, and baking at high heat can lead to the formation of acrylamide, the levels formed vary widely among different products and between production lots of the same food products. One fact, however, is clear: The information so far indicates that boiling food does not lead to measurable acrylamide formation. Luckily, as you will learn later in this book, there are also several other wonderful cooking methods and strategies that will prevent acrylamide formation, including cooking with liquids, as in poaching and steaming, and marinating food before cooking.

In the next chapter, you will discover how to recognize and therefore avoid foods that promote the AGEs that are dangerous to your mind, body, and appearance.

2

Finding the AGEs in Your Food

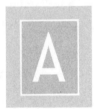ccording to Drs. Melpomeni Peppa, Helen Vlassara, and Jaime Uribarri, writing in *Clinical Diabetes*, the journal of the American Diabetes Association, a significant proportion—as much as 10%—of AGEs is absorbed with food. The rest is formed inside the body as described on pages 8–10.

Another study, published in the *Journal of Geronotology: Medical Sciences* in April 2007, was even more alarming. It showed that in all the participants, the more AGE-rich food they ate, the more AGEs were found in their blood, and the higher their levels of markers of inflammation. In addition, researchers found that those participants who were 65 and older had AGE levels 35% higher than those participants who were 45 or younger.

Most troubling of all is that the *Clinical Diabetes* study showed that some of the younger healthy adults had AGE levels on par with diabetic patients in earlier studies! That led Vlassara, the lead author of the study, to state that food processors should put AGE levels on nutrition labels so that buyers could consider their AGE intake the same way they do trans fats and sodium levels. I have now taken up this cause as well. In fact, I wrote this book to bring AGEs to the public arena so that consumers and government agencies alike can demand that AGEs in foods be listed and eliminated wherever possible.

What this tells us is that reducing and/or eliminating AGEs in the diet is an important health, anti-aging, and anti-inflammatory strategy. Unfortunately, most people have no idea that AGEs even exist, let alone are copiously added to processed foods. That's why we all have to learn how to read food and beverage labels so that we can recognize hidden forms of AGEs. When you read a label, make sure you understand what each ingredient is. If you don't know what an ingredient is, it is better to avoid the product.

FOOD ADDITIVES TO AVOID

Hidden Sugars Sugar comes in many forms. As you might assume, when we eat sugar, it raises our blood-sugar level, and chronically high blood-sugar levels lead to the creation of the sugar bonds known as AGEs. Therefore, it is very important to recognize that there are many forms of sugar; in fact, the word "sugar" may not appear on a label at all. Look for white sugar, cane sugar, brown sugar, confectioner's sugar, invert sugar, raw sugar, beet sugar, turbinado sugar, corn syrup, high-fructose corn syrup, dextrin, honey, maple, evaporated cane juice, malt, molasses, dextrose, fructose, sucrose, fruit juice concentrate, glucose, and maltose.

Artificial Coloring Synthetic food dyes are unnecessary, and are either toxic or possible carcinogens, which means that they may promote cancer.

Aspartame and All Artificial Sweeteners, Including Saccharin These are dangerous excitotoxins with many negative effects.

BHT and BHA These are used to preserve fats and oils. Studies indicate that they may be carcinogenic.

Brominated Vegetable Oil (BVO) This is used in citrus-flavored sodas and is banned in more than 100 countries. It has been linked to damage in the major organ systems. Apparently the FDA does not require that it be listed on labels—so avoid any citrus-flavored sodas (such as lemon or lime), as it is a good bet that BVO is included.

Carrageenan This is a stabilizer and thickening agent found in everything from ice cream to yogurt. It may be a carcinogen, and is linked to such conditions as ulcers and cancer. In addition to suppressing immune function, carrageenan causes intestinal ulcers and inflammatory bowel disease in animals, and some research indicates that carrageenan is associated with causing cancer in humans.

Partially Hydrogenated Vegetable Oils These are the infamous trans fats, directly linked to heart disease. The FDA published a paper stating that if people in the U.S. stopped eating trans fat there would be 30,000 to 100,000 fewer deaths per year from coronary heart disease (CHD). Trans fats are also linked to breast and colon cancer, atherosclerosis, elevated cholesterol, depressed immune systems, and allergies.

Nitrates These form powerful cancer-causing agents in the stomach. They are found in smoked foods such as deli foods, cured meats, bacon, hot dogs, pepperoni, and sausage.

Monosodium Glutamate (MSG) This is a dangerous excitotoxin that may cause headaches, itching, nausea, nervous system and reproductive disorders, and high blood pressure. Pregnant and lactating mothers, infants, and small children should avoid MSG. Allergic reactions are common. MSG may be hidden in Chinese food, infant formula, low-fat milk, candy, chewing gum, drinks, and over-the-counter medications. Look for the following ingredients that are or contain MSG:

Monosodium Glutamate	Hydrolyzed Plant Protein
Hydrolyzed Vegetable Protein	Calcium Caseinate
Hydrolyzed Protein	Sodium Caseinate

Yeast Extract	Hydrolyzed Oat Flour
Textured Protein (Including TVP)	Autolyzed Yeast
Plant Protein Extract	Corn Oil

Neotame This is related to aspartame, but is allegedly more toxic.

Olestra This fat substitute causes gastrointestinal distress. It also lowers absorption of carotenoids (nutrients that lower our risk of cancer) and other fat-soluble nutrients.

Potassium Bromate Bromate causes cancer. Potassium bromate is used in bread making.

Sulfites These can cause dangerous allergic reactions.

COMMON FOOD SOURCES OF AGES INCLUDE:

- All foods that are cooked at high heats;

- Foods cooked at low heats for long periods with no liquid;

- Charbroiled meats;

- Roasted meats;

- Rotisserie chickens, turkeys, etc. Browned poultry skin is a significant source of AGEs.

- Fried foods;

- Roasted or toasted nuts and seeds;

- Prepackaged baked goods that are deep brown in color usually signify the addition of sugars or caramel coloring, making them a source of exogenous AGEs.

- Processed snack (or "junk") foods (potato chips, pretzels, etc.);

- Fast foods (Most fast food outlets offer fare that is rife with trans fats, charbroiled meats, fried foods, and soft drinks);

■ Coffee (In addition to raising levels of the stress hormone cortisol, coffee beans are dark roasted, fostering the formation of AGEs); and

■ All forms of soda. Soda is dangerous for several reasons, including its sugar content and, even worse, its high-fructose corn syrup. In fact, almost every bottle or can of soda on the market is made with high-fructose corn syrup, which increases the appetite and promotes obesity to a far greater degree than cane sugar. A great many sodas also contain caramel coloring, not just the obvious ones, such as colas and root beer. Sodas can also contain sodium benzoate, a popular preservative that can react with ascorbic acid to form the cancer-causing chemical benzene.

The Color of AGEs

Just thinking of caramel makes many people's mouths water. But caramel coloring, a popular coloring in sodas such as colas and many other foods, is actually burned sugar, which is both carcinogenic and immunosuppressive. The FDA is aware of this, and mandates that any food or beverage containing caramel coloring must list it on the product label. Unfortunately, most people are not aware of this darker side to a substance that sounds harmless but is in fact toxic. Caramel coloring is also a source of exogenous AGEs. When combined with the sugar and/or high-fructose corn syrup found in sodas, we are getting a double dose of AGEs. Drink a cola along with a heaping plate of French fries and a charbroiled, grilled hamburger doused with high-fructose corn syrup–sweetened ketchup—well, I think you get the picture. This popular combination is a serious contributor to accelerated aging and AGE formation in all organ systems. This is important for children as well because AGEs accumulate with age and foods like this mean that they will get an early start in age-accelerating glycating compounds.

GROWING AGE-RELATED EPIDEMICS

As the world's population both increases and ages, the number of people who are affected by AGE-related diseases increases as well. Finding successful therapeutic strategies to combat Alzheimer's disease, dementia, and diabetes has never been more important than it is today.

It's a Mad, Mad, Mad World

If you sometimes think that the whole world has gone crazy, you may not be too far off the mark. A study entitled "Global Prevalence of Dementia: A Delphi Consensus Study" (C.P. Ferri et al.) estimated that 24 million people worldwide have Alzheimer's disease or some other form of dementia, with one new case every seven seconds (4.6 million new cases every year). And that is not the only bad news. It is estimated that the number of people affected may double every 20 years. The authors said that in 2001, some 60% of dementia cases occurred in developing countries, and that this proportion may rise to 71% by 2040.

A major culprit in the rise of Alzheimer's disease and other forms of dementia is the adoption of the Western lifestyle by developing countries. As our ubiquitous "fast" and "convenience" foods pop up around the world with increasing frequency, they are taking the place of natural, healthy native cuisines. The number of dementia cases occurring in their populations is forecast to increase 100% by 2040, and to increase more than 300% in India, China, and their immediate neighbors.

Although longer life spans contribute to Alzheimer's disease, many observers attribute the rapid worldwide rise in dementia rates to the increasing dominance of the standard Western diet, which is low in protective dietary factors (fish-derived omega-3 fatty acids, fiber, and plant-derived antioxidants). In place of these life and health benefits, Western foods are high in fat, sugar, and calories—making these foods high in AGE-forming properties as well. And AGE formation plays a significant role in Alzheimer's disease. Fighting AGEs and the related inflammation is the best strategy we have to combat this disease.

It is not just Alzheimer's disease that is increasing in epidemic proportions. According to the World Health Organization, an estimated 30 million people worldwide had diabetes in 1985. A decade later, the global burden of diabetes was estimated to be 135 million. The latest WHO estimate for the number of people with diabetes worldwide in 2000 is 171 million. This is likely to increase to at least 366 million by 2030. Two major concerns are that much of this increase in diabetes will occur in developing countries (due to population growth, aging, unhealthy diets, obesity, and sedentary lifestyles) and that there is a growing incidence of type 2 diabetes—which accounts for about 90% of all cases—at younger ages. In developed countries most people with diabetes are above the age of retirement. In developing countries those most frequently affected are in the middle, productive years of their lives, between 35 and 64.

Insulin Resistance: Beyond Diabetes

There is a tremendous focus on diabetes today, due in large part to the obesity epidemic and the alarmingly increased occurrence of insulin resistance in children (heretofore unheard-of) and adults. Insulin is a hormone released by the pancreas in response to increased levels of sugar in the blood. Insulin resistance occurs when the insulin receptors on our cells lose sensitivity and fail to utilize insulin effectively. To compensate for the body's muted reaction to insulin, more insulin is produced in an effort to reduce glucose levels. Simply put, when we are insulin resistant, our insulin mechanism does not work as well as it should. This condition leads to elevated insulin levels, leading to insulin resistance. The high levels of circulating glucose can become chemically attached to proteins and DNA, and are thought to play an important role in the aging process through increased formation of free radicals, damage to the DNA, and, of course, AGEs.

Many scientists, including Harry Preuss, M.D. at Georgetown University, believe that because of its AGE-accelerating properties, insulin resistance reaches way beyond diabetes to play a prominent role in the rate of aging. Common age-related disorders such as cardiovascular diseases, obesity, and cancer are, in fact, generally recognized to be linked to insulin resistance. In addition, insulin resistance is often found in the elderly, and has been linked to the aging process in carefully controlled animal studies. Disturbed glucose/insulin metabolism may also adversely influence bone metabolism and the onset and progression of tumor formation and growth—again, problems commonly found in aging.

Many well-controlled animal and human studies show that heavy sugar ingestion results in insulin resistance from chronically high levels of insulin circulating in the blood. This condition can lead to metabolic syndrome, a dangerous quartet of metabolic imbalances that increase the risk of both cardiovascular disease and diabetes:

1. high blood pressure;

2. elevated levels of insulin;

3. excess weight (especially around the abdomen); and

4. dyslipidemia, meaning low levels of HDL (good cholesterol), high levels of LDL (bad cholesterol), and high levels of triglycerides (metabolized dietary fats that end up in our blood, organs, and tissues).

There is also a large body of evidence linking glucose intolerance and insulin resistance to an increased risk of coronary artery disease (CAD). One of the potential mechanisms by which hyperglycemia (high blood sugar levels) may contribute to CAD is through the formation of AGEs. According to a groundbreaking study published in the September 2001 issue of *Diabetes Care*, "Advanced Glycation End Products in Nondiabetic Patients with Coronary Artery Disease" by Drs. Kanauchi, Tsujimoto, and Hashimoto, AGE formation may lead to oxidative stress, which may lead to insulin resistance. And as you will learn in later chapters, atherosclerosis, a major cause of heart disease and stroke, is mediated by AGEs.

Scientists are finding increased medical complications from the formation of AGEs in both diabetics and the general aging population. Because of the increased availability of glucose in diabetics, this glycation formation is markedly accelerated. Consequently, those with uncontrolled diabetes age one third faster than nondiabetics!

We know that the ubiquitous sugar, high-fructose corn syrup, fast and processed foods, and refined starches in the Western diet are major contributors to metabolic syndrome and AGE formation—as is the lack of healthy fats, fresh fruits and vegetables, and fiber, all of which can help mitigate the negative effects of AGE-producing foods.

This is the bad news. The good news is that in the chapters that follow I apply the three-tiered formula of diet, supplements, and topicals, each of which is designed to work synergistically to stop the destructive power of AGEs. You will learn cooking methods that do not promote the formation of AGEs, and discover a remarkable substance that safely blocks the digestion of carbohydrates—allowing us to occasionally have our cake and eat it too.

PART TWO

Food That
Fights AGEs

3

The Anti-AGEs Diet

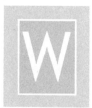

hether we are talking about weight problems, wrinkles, or serious disease, we know that AGEs are major causative factors. In fact, as Perricone readers know, and numerous scientific studies bear out, inflammation, which is at the very basis of AGE formation, is implicated in aging and age-related diseases.

Our daily food choices play significant roles in how well or poorly we are aging, both internally and externally. Fortunately for us, as you will learn later in this chapter, certain foods are unsurpassed in keeping our cells functioning at optimum levels, offering us our best protection against the AGE accelerators that cause us to be susceptible to diabetes, heart disease, cancer, and other related degenerative diseases.

EAT WELL TO LIVE WELL

Our food choices as well as our methods of food preparation are of paramount importance for preventing AGEs. When we cook high-glycemic carbohydrates (that is, carbs that rapidly convert to sugar when eaten), protein, and/or fat at elevated temperatures, we are generating high levels of AGEs. However, it is important to clarify that not all carbohydrates are implicated. The majority of vegetables and whole grains will not rapidly convert to sugar in the bloodstream when eaten, so they are not generally worrisome sources of AGEs. Unlike most vegetables, potatoes are high glycemic. If they are cooked in hot oil (as French fries and potato chips are) they become significant sources of AGEs as well as the toxic acrylamide discussed in Chapter One.

Foods that naturally have higher fat levels generate more AGEs. In general, low-fat, high-fiber foods, including legumes, other vegetables, and grains, tend to be low in AGEs. That said, if you fry a veggie or nut burger at high heats, you will be promoting the formation of AGEs. Nuts and seeds, which have a naturally high fat content, can become sources of AGEs when they are roasted. To enjoy the health benefits of nuts and seeds, eat them in their raw state.

This chapter contains extensive food lists in all of the important categories to help you make the right choices, as well as many delicious recipes and tips on correct food preparation—a key strategy to prevent AGE formation.

The Right Way to Cook

We now know that cooking foods at high temperatures, or at low temperatures for extended periods, generates significant AGEs. It does not matter whether the food is grilled, roasted, fried, broiled, barbecued, microwaved, or sautéed. It is the heat—high or lengthy—that counts.

A study from the *Proceedings of the National Academy of Sciences* showed that consuming foods high in AGEs might be responsible for the induction of a low-grade but chronic state of inflammation. In addition, the AGEs created when food is cooked at high temperatures also promote the formation of AGEs in our living tissues.

The implications of these findings are profound. They inspire us to rethink what we eat and how we prepare it. The *National Academy* scientists observed that cooking and aging have similar biological properties. Cooking foods at high temperatures results in a "browning" effect, in which the sugars and certain oxidized fats react with proteins to form AGEs in the food. The article also stated that normal aging can be regarded as a slow cooking process, since these same AGEs form in the skin, arteries, eye lenses, joints, cartilage, and other places in our bodies. Scientists have known of these dangers for years; unfortunately, it appears to have been a well-kept secret not apparent to the average person.

In the study noted in Chapter Two, Drs. Peppa, Vlassara, and Uribarri found not only that we absorb about 10% of AGEs from foods, but also that only one third of what is absorbed is excreted within 48 hours in the urine of people with normal kidney function. AGEs that are not excreted are deposited in tissues, where they remain biologically active, posing a serious threat. Diabetics, who frequently have kidney (renal) impairment, are at an increased risk for AGE formation and the resulting damage. However, as we age, nondiabetics also see an increase in AGE formation, and are at greater risk for AGE-related diseases and disorders.

Liquid Magic

If the thought of a lifetime of eating boiled or steamed chicken is less than appealing, take heart. Adding moisture to the cooking process will significantly lower the formation of AGEs, and actually make food taste better if prepared correctly. Remember, glycation is a *browning reaction.* When we deeply brown meats and other foods, charring or blackening them over dry heat and high temperatures, we are creating exogenous AGEs. Cooking with moisture will alleviate this. A well-done grilled steak is like shoe leather thanks to the cross-linking of the proteins with the fats. A gently poached piece of fish is moist and supple because it is not creating AGEs (see Chapter Eleven for examples of cooking proteins that will not promote AGE formation).

Although it is wise to limit your intake of red meats (unless you have access to organic, grass-fed varieties as opposed to grain fed), you can still enjoy them occasionally without accelerating AGE development. Your best bets for cooking are to include some form of liquid, such as making a savory soup or stew with broth or tomatoes. Another great strategy is to marinate protein foods (meats and tofu) prior to cooking. Flavor is greatly enhanced when foods are prepared with a tasty marinade. Even barbecued ribs (trim excess fat) can be enjoyed occasionally when marinated and slow cooked in a sauce over low heat. Do not coat your meat or tofu in flour, which is a high-glycemic food that will increase AGE formation. If you want to coat it with something, grind up fresh nuts or seeds.

AGE-Less Barbecuing

If you choose to barbecue, cut your meat or vegetables into small pieces (as in preparing shish kabobs). This will allow the food to cook much more quickly, even over low heat, and prevent the AGE formation that comes from long cooking times. Obviously, there are times when this will not work, like when you're cooking the Thanksgiving turkey. If Thanksgiving was the only time you had an AGE-packed meal, it would not be a problem. Unfortunately, ingesting AGEs is more like a three-time-a-day occurrence. The point here is to raise awareness of how AGEs form during the cooking process. This will enable us to scale back on the cooking methods that promote their formation.

The Right Fats in the Right Amounts

As you now know, eating even healthful foods cooked at high temperatures results in the formation of AGEs. A general rule of thumb is to keep your saturated fat intake to no more than 10% of your total caloric intake. Saturated fats are found in meats and dairy products. High-saturated-fat intake is linked to insulin resistance, which is, in turn, linked to inflammation and AGEs. You can lower your intake of saturated fat by choosing leaner cuts of meat (like the aforementioned grass-fed beef) and by substituting extra-virgin olive oil for butter whenever possible.

When it comes to the types of fats found in salmon and other types of seafood (omega-3s), the news is good—these fats actually reduce insulin resistance and help keep the blood vessels and arteries healthy and supple. The fats that occur naturally in foods such as nuts, olives, olive oil, and avocados are also beneficial. The Mediterranean diet, which is high in fish, olive oil, and the other healthy sources of fat listed above, is well known for its role in promoting cardiovascular health.

The Best Carbs for the Job

The importance of complex carbohydrates—such as those found naturally in fresh fruits and vegetables, beans and lentils, and whole grains—really cannot be overemphasized in AGE prevention. Not only are they rich in anti-inflammatory antioxidants, they also contain multiple disease-preventing phytonutrients and all-important fiber. Fiber-rich foods slow down the digestive process and prevent the rapid release of glucose in the bloodstream.

The standard American diet is seriously low in fiber, which helps account for people's tendency to overeat, because fiber slows digestion, helping us to feel full longer. A diet low in fiber also contributes to disturbances in blood sugar and insulin. Fiber can help prevent kidney and gallstones, as well as certain types of cancer, including breast, ovarian, colon, and uterine cancer. According to the National Institutes of Health, the average American now eats 10 to 15 grams of fiber per day. The recommendation for older children, adolescents, and adults is 20 to 35 grams per day. Younger children will not be able to eat enough calories to achieve this, but introducing whole grains, fresh fruits, and other high-fiber foods is suggested.

To ensure adequate fiber intake, eat a variety of foods (fruits and vegetables, including dried beans and peas, whole grains and cereals). Add fiber gradually over a period of a few weeks to avoid abdominal discomfort. Water aids the passage of fiber through the digestive system, so drink plenty of fluids (approximately eight glasses of water or noncaloric fluid a day).

Peeling the skin off fruits and vegetables will reduce their fiber content. This is why it is important to purchase organic fruits and vegetables. You will then be able to safely eat the skin of the food after washing it thoroughly. Eating the skin of nonorganic fruits and vegetables is not recommended because of possible toxic pesticide residue.

Cooking may actually increase your fiber intake by decreasing the volume of the food. For example, when you steam or sauté spinach you can eat a larger amount of the vegetable, thereby getting more fiber. If you put a pound of cooked spinach next to a pound of raw spinach you'll see what I mean—the cooked spinach is about ¼ the volume. Just don't overcook the vegetables. A quick sauté is ideal for greens like spinach, while steaming is perfect for asparagus and broccoli. Eat plenty of uncooked fruits and vegetables as well, because the raw foods contain important enzymes that are lost in the cooking process.

Soluble fiber, such as the beta glucans found in oats, attracts water during digestion and slows the rate of nutrient absorption. It helps prevent heart disease by exerting a positive effect on cholesterol, triglycerides, and other particles in the blood. Soluble fiber also helps us feel full so that we automatically eat less. Fiber also slows the absorption of carbohydrates, resulting in the lowering of the glycemic index of specific foods. High-fiber diets can also increase insulin sensitivity, and are indispensable components in preventing AGE formation.

Food Sources of Fiber

The following is a list of the fiber content of many popular fruits, vegetables, nuts, and seeds. Keep in mind that only foods from the plant world contain fiber—there is no fiber in meat. Because of the complexity of fruits and vegetables, scientists have not been able to determine their exact amount of fiber, so all amounts are approximations.

Food Sources of Fiber

FOOD	PORTION	CALORIES	FIBER (GRAMS)
Almonds			
slivered	1 tbsp	14	0.6
sliced	¼ cup	56	2.4
Apples			
raw	1 small	55–60	3.0
raw	1 med	70	4.0
raw	1 large	80–100	4.5
Apricots			
raw	1 whole	17	0.8
dried	2 halves	36	1.7

FOOD	PORTION	CALORIES	FIBER (GRAMS)
Artichokes			
cooked	1 large	30–44	4.5
canned hearts	4 or 5 sm	24	4.5
Asparagus			
cooked, small spears	½ cup	17	1.7
Avocados			
diced	¼ cup	97	1.7
sliced	2 slices	50	0.9
whole	½ avg.	170	2.8
Bananas	1 med 8″	96	3.0
Barley			
hulled	¼ cup dry	110	4.0
Beans			
black, cooked	1 cup	190	19.4
broad beans (Italian, haricot canned or cooked)	¾ cup	30	3.0
Great Northern (canned or cooked)	1 cup	160	16.0
kidney beans, canned	½ cup	94	9.7
lima, Fordhook baby, butter beans (canned or cooked)	½ cup	118	3.7
lima, dried canned or cooked	½ cup	150	5.8
pinto, dried before cooking	½ cup	155	18.8
canned or cooked	1 cup	155	18.8
white, dried before cooking	½ cup	160	16.0
canned or cooked	½ cup	80	8.0

FOOD	PORTION	CALORIES	FIBER (GRAMS)

(See also **chickpeas, Green [snap] beans, lentils, and peas.**)

Bean sprouts, raw

in salad	¼ cup	7	0.8

Beet greens, cooked (see Greens, cooked)

Blackberries

raw, no sugar	½ cup	27	4.4

Brazil nuts

shelled	2	48	2.5

Broccoli

raw	½ cup	20	4.0
frozen	4 spears	20	5.0
fresh, cooked	¾ cup	30	7.0

Brussels sprouts

cooked	¾ cup	36	3.0

Buckwheat groats (kasha)

before cooking	½ cup	160	9.6
cooked	1 cup	160	9.6

Cabbage, white or red

raw	½ cup	8	1.5
cooked	⅔ cup	15	3.0

Cantaloupes

	¼	38	1.0

Carrots

raw, slivered (4-5 sticks)	¼ cup	10	1.7
cooked	½ cup	20	3.4

FOOD	PORTION	CALORIES	FIBER (GRAMS)
Cauliflower			
raw, chopped	3 tiny buds	10	1.2
cooked, chopped	⅞ cup	16	2.3
Celery, Pascal			
raw	¼ cup	5	2.0
chopped	2 tbsp.	3	1.0
cooked	½ cup	9	3.0
Cherries	10	28	1.2
sweet, raw	½ cup	55	1.0
Chestnuts			
roasted	2 lg	29	1.9
Chickpeas (garbanzos)			
canned	½ cup	86	6.0
cooked	1 cup	172	12.0
Coconut, dried			
unsweetened	1 tbsp	22	3.4
Cranberries			
raw	¼ cup	12	2.0
Cucumber, raw			
unpeeled	10 thin sl	12	0.7
Eggplant			
baked with tomatoes	2 thick sl	42	4.0
Endive, raw			
salad	10 leaves	10	0.6
Grapefruit	½ avg	30	0.8

FOOD	PORTION	CALORIES	FIBER (GRAMS)
Grapes			
white	20	75	1.0
red or black	15–20	65	1.0
Green (snap) beans			
fresh or frozen	½ cup	10	2.1
Greens, cooked			
collards, beet greens, dandelion, kale, Swiss chard, turnip greens	½ cup	20	4.0
Honeydew melon	3″ slice	42	1.5
Lentils			
brown, raw	⅓ cup	144	5.5
brown, cooked	⅔ cup	144	5.5
red, raw	½ cup	192	6.4
red, cooked	1 cup	192	6.4
Lettuce			
(Boston, leaf, iceberg) shredded	1 cup	5	0.8
Mushrooms			
raw	5 sm	4	1.4
sauteed or baked with 2 tsp diet margarine	4 lg	45	2.0
canned sliced, water-packed	¼ cup	10	2.0
Oatmeal (old fashioned)	½ cup dry	150	4.0
Okra			
fresh or frozen, cooked	½ cup	13	1.6

FOOD	PORTION	CALORIES	FIBER (GRAMS)
Olives			
green	6	42	1.2
black	6	96	1.2
Onion			
raw	1 tbsp	4	0.2
cooked	½ cup	22	1.5
green, raw (scallion)	¼ cup	11	0.8
Oranges	1 lg	70	2.4
	1 sm	35	1.2
Parsley, chopped	2 tbsp	4	0.6
	1 tbsp	2	0.3
Parsnip, pared			
cooked	1 lg	76	2.8
	1 sm	38	1.4
Peaches			
raw	1 med	38	2.3
Pears	1 med	88	4.0
Peas			
green, fresh or frozen	½ cup	60	9.1
black-eyed frozen/canned	½ cup	74	8.0
split peas, dried	½ cup	63	6.7
cooked	1 cup	126	13.4
(See also **Chickpeas**)			
Peas and carrots			
frozen	½ package (5 oz)	40	6.2

FOOD	PORTION	CALORIES	FIBER (GRAMS)
Peppers			
green sweet, raw	2 tbsp	4	0.3
green sweet, cooked	½ cup	13	1.2
red sweet (pimento)	2 tbsp.	9	1.0
red chili, fresh	1 tbsp.	7	1.2
dried, crushed	1 tsp	7	1.2
Pimento (see Peppers)			
Pineapple			
fresh, cubed	½ cup	41	0.8
canned	1 cup	58–74	0.8
Plums	2 or 3 sm	38–45	2.0
Sweet Potatoes			
baked or boiled	1 sm (5 oz)	146	4.0
Radishes	3	5	0.1
Raspberries, red			
fresh/frozen	½ cup	20	4.6
Rutabaga (yellow turnip)	½ cup	40	3.2
Spinach			
raw	1 cup	8	3.5
cooked	½ cup	26	7.0
Split peas (see Peas)			
Squash			
summer (yellow)	½ cup	8	2.0
winter, baked or mashed	½ cup	40–50	3.5
Zucchini, raw or cooked	½ cup	7	3.0

FOOD	PORTION	CALORIES	FIBER (GRAMS)
Strawberries	1 cup	45	3.0
Tomatoes			
raw	1 sm	22	1.4
canned	½ cup	21	1.0
sauce	½ cup	20	0.5
Turnips, white			
raw, slivered	¼ cup	8	1.2
cooked	½ cup	16	2.0
Watercress			
raw	½ cup (20 sprigs)	4	1.0
Watermelon	1 thick slice	68	2.8
Yams			
cooked or baked in skin	1 med (6 oz.)	156	6.8

Eat Fish, Live Longer

As noted, scientists have confirmed that AGEs are causative factors in cardiovascular disease. Just as the sugars in an onion will caramelize when cooked for a long period, as we age our organs can also caramelize. An example of this is the uncontrolled diabetic, whose body has high levels of AGEs. This places these diabetics at a greater risk for kidney disease, and it is well documented that kidney disease increases the risk of heart disease. In fact, most patients with kidney disease actually die of complications from heart disease rather than kidney failure. This provides even more impetus to decrease the development of AGEs, because statistics estimate that close to 70% of diabetics will die from heart disease or stroke. And while there is not a solid scientific body of evidence proving that omega-3 essential fatty acids help prevent kidney disease in

An Extraordinary Disease Predictor

Excessive C-reactive protein (CRP) in the blood is a biomarker for systemic inflammation. Thus CRP is also a biomarker for metabolic syndrome, type 2 diabetes, hypertension, and cardiovascular disease (CVD), and is directly linked to body mass—that is, how much we weigh, because inflammation is elevated in all these processes. In addition, CRP upregulates receptors for AGE products in human endothelial cells, which line the inside of some body cavities, including blood vessels. This means that CRP *increases* the number of receptors for AGEs on cell surfaces, making them perfect targets for the damaging effects of AGEs.

Elevated CRP is also an extraordinarily accurate predictor of atherosclerosis, which is the clogging, narrowing, and hardening of the blood vessels. In fact, measuring CRP is much more accurate than measuring cholesterol as a predictor of atherosclerosis. Atherosclerosis can lead to stroke, heart attack, eye problems, and kidney problems.

CRP levels can be lowered with physical activity; anti-inflammatory drugs such as aspirin; antioxidant supplements, including alpha lipoic acid and Vitamin C; foods high in antioxidants and fiber such as fresh fruits and vegetables; omega-3 essential fatty acids; and weight loss in obese individuals.

In addition, wild salmon, my favorite food, also has a very positive effect on CRP because of its powerful anti-inflammatory properties. This is partly due to the presence of omega-3 essential fatty acids, which are also available in high-quality fish-oil capsules (more about this in Chapter Four).

humans the way they appear to in dogs, there is solid evidence that they can prevent heart disease.

Thanks to their anti-inflammatory properties, the long-chain marine omega-3s (DHA and EPA) concentrated in fatty fish such as salmon, tuna, sablefish, and sardines appear to rival the life-saving powers of statins, the most effective drugs yet found for preventing heart attacks.

While we are well aware that fish and marine omega-3s significantly reduce the risk of heart attack and stroke, we've lacked direct evidence showing that they do so by reducing the kinds of AGE-generated inflammation increasingly accepted (along with high cholesterol levels) as key risk factors for heart attack.

That important data gap has now been bridged, thanks to new research from the ongoing ATTICA study in Greece, named for that famous city, which involves 1,514 healthy men and 1,528 healthy women living in and around Athens, Greece. Researchers are examining these people to determine the role of several dietary and lifestyle factors in raising or lowering the risk of heart disease.

About 90% of the ATTICA study participants reported eating fish at least once a month. Compared with those who ate little fish, the participants who ate the most fish—about 10.5 ounces per week—had much lower levels of five key markers of inflammation—as much as 33% lower! The Greek researchers also found significantly lower levels of these inflammation markers in participants who ate between five and ten ounces of fish per week.

The researchers were careful to adjust for other factors that might influence inflammation, including demographic and socioeconomic variables, smoking, blood pressure, cholesterol levels, and diabetes. The scientific team concluded that "fish consumption was independently associated with lower inflammatory markers among healthy adults. The strength and consistency of this finding has [sic] implications for public health and should be explored further."

Study coauthor Demosthenes Panagiotakos, Ph.D., in an interview with the American College of Cardiology, said that these results support existing medical advice that people should eat more fish, particularly the types of oily fish that have high levels of omega-3 fatty acids. "For the general public it could be suggested that consuming fish one or two times per week could lead to these beneficial effects found in our study," said Panagiotakos. "The general recommendation is to avoid frying the fish. Local small fish (like sardines) which usually is [sic] consumed with the bone are good sources of omega-3 fatty acids."

Lead author Antonis Zampelas, Ph.D. added that the results indicate that logically, omega-3 supplements should be comparably beneficial. "We revealed that not only the fish portion, but also the amount of omega-3 fatty acids seems to play a role in the reduction of inflammatory marker levels," said Zampelas. "Therefore we can speculate that omega-3 fatty acid intake in the level of 0.6 grams (600 mg) per day could be applicable to other populations, irrespective of the source of fish."

This is more proof that salmon is one of the greatest health-promoting, anti-aging foods available. A special note about wild salmon: Unlike many wild fish, salmon is a sustainable food. According to information from Vital Choice Seafood, Alaska's wild salmon runs are among the healthiest on earth. Each year, tens of millions of Alaska salmon return to spawn in their natal rivers. Pristine habitat and well-managed commercial fisheries contribute to the preservation of Alaska's most precious sustainable natural resource. Alaskan salmon have the distinction of becoming the first U.S. fish to be certified sustainable by the Marine Stewardship Council Environmental Standard. Excellent wild salmon also hails from Canada and California.

A Special Note on *Fish*

Fish and seafood are traditionally low in fat, and do not cause or contain AGEs unless you deep-fry them in batter. Remember, it is foods that are high in sugar and saturated fats that are the problem. High-fat fish, such as salmon, trout, sardines, herring, anchovies, and trout, contain healthy fats and do not contain the saturated fat found in beef, lamb, and other meats.

That said, high heat will turn your fish into a rubbery, unappealing state. Always cook fish gently; poaching or lightly sautéing are ideal. And whatever you do, skip heavily fried and breaded fish and chips, which pose a triple AGE whammy from the batter, the high heat, and the frying. See Chapter Eleven for appetizing recipes.

GOING GREEN: BENEFITS OF A PLANT-RICH DIET

Because AGEs are such important generators of oxidative stress and free radicals, resulting in a highly destructive inflammatory cascade, and because they increase in our bodies with each passing year, we need very targeted nutritional strategies to combat their effects. I have found that what are commonly known as "green foods" provide an exceptional concentration of anti-inflammatory, AGE-preventing antioxidants. Unfortunately, no matter how good our intentions, it can be difficult to consume the level of fresh fruits and vegetables needed for optimum health and protection from the ravages of both aging and AGEs. However, research continues to recognize the importance of a plant-rich diet, in conjunction with high-quality sources of protein.

Experts agree that a diet lacking in essential vitamins creates a greater risk for a degenerative disease. While most people in the United States are aware of the importance of regular consumption of fruits and vegetables for preventing diseases like diabetes, cardiovascular disease, and cancer, surveys indicate that fewer than 40% consume even the lowest recommended three to five combined servings per day. And even that recommended number might be too low, as Americans who eat seven or more servings of fruits and vegetables daily reduce the risk of heart disease and cancer by more than 50%.

The nutritional excellence of green foods has been well documented for decades, and for good reason: Green foods, including young barley grass, contain an abundance of essential nutrients and beneficial phytonutrients, including flavonoids, carotenoids, catechins, and chlorophyll.

If one studies the research literature on the health benefits of fruits and vegetables, it is clear that both amount and variety are important. Until recently, nutrition experts believed that the health benefits of plants were derived from their constituent macronutrients (carbohydrates, fats, protein, and fiber) and micronutrients (vitamins and minerals). But it is now clear that although these nutrients are essential, many of the disease-preventing qualities of plants can be attributed to specific phytonutrients, thousands of which have already been identified. While it may be impractical for many people to consume even a small portion of thousands of individual phytonutrients, we may still reap their collective benefits by including in our diets a variety of the plants that contain the known types of phytonutrients. Some of these phytonutrients and foods that contain them are:

Phytonutrients and Their Sources

PHYTONUTRIENT TYPE	FOODS
Allyl sulfur compounds:	garlic, onions
Anthocyanidins:	blackberries, blueberries, grapes, raspberries
Carotenoids:	carrots, yams, pumpkin
Catechins:	green tea, grapes, leafy greens
Coumarins:	green vegetables, citrus fruits
Glucosinolates:	broccoli, Brussels sprouts, kale, cabbage
Isoflavones:	soy, kudzu, red clover, flax, rye
Isoflavonoids:	barley grass, wheat grass, leafy greens
Lignans:	flax, rye
Limonoids:	citrus fruits
Phenolic acids:	berries, cherries, grapes, citrus fruits
Phytosterols:	soybeans
Tocopherols and tocotrienols:	whole grains

In addition to providing these known types of phytonutrients, a diet containing many different types of plants will include beneficial phytonutrients not yet identified. Since eating a varied diet may be prove to be difficult for many people, the Green Foods Corporation has developed the whole-food, multi-ingredient dietary supplement Green Magma®, in order to supply those beneficial phytonutrients that may be missing from our diet. Green Magma contains a base of barley grass juice powder (1,800 mg per serving) and other natural ingredients that includes concentrated powdered extracts of fruits, vegetables, herbs, probiotics, and digestive enzymes. The last three ingredients were added to promote good digestion and nutrient absorption. For my own regimen, I take both Green Magma and Veggie Magma (see page 44) every day. The powerful anti-inflammatory antioxidants in these products provide a very targeted antidote to AGE formation and AGE prevention.

Young Barley Grass

Barley grass is one of the premier green foods researched extensively by Green Foods Corporation's founder, Yoshihide Hagiwara, M.D. Research by Dr. Hagiwara and others at leading universities has clearly demonstrated the health benefits of barley grass, which include increased energy levels, enhanced digestion and immunity, cardiovascular support, anti-inflammatory actions, antioxidant protection, and the breakdown of organophosphate pesticides.

Barley grass is alkaline, and is abundant in vitamins, minerals, amino acids, and active enzymes. Its deep green color is due to its large amount of natural chlorophyll, a well-known cleanser and deodorizer. Superoxide dismutase, an enzyme important in neutralizing inflammation-inducing free radicals in our cells, is also found in large amounts in barley grass. Barley grass is also rich in potassium, calcium, and magnesium, and by weight it has more vitamin C than oranges and more iron than spinach.

Green Magma provides our bodies with a natural whole-food source of vitamins, minerals, proteins, essential and nonessential amino acids, active enzymes, antioxidants, detoxifiers, and chlorophyll. Since Green Magma contains essential nutrients and all the major types of phytonutrients, it will help nourish and protect the entire body.

But how does the nutrient content of Green Magma compare to that of fresh whole vegetables? In other words, are you really receiving the nutritional equivalent of several servings or more of fresh vegetables by taking Green Magma?

To answer this question, the nutritional content of single servings of fresh, raw garden vegetables such as alfalfa, broccoli, cabbage, carrots, cauliflower, cucumbers, lettuce, spinach, and tomatoes were compared to those found in single servings of Green Magma. The nutrient data for Green Magma and the vegetables are based on certified nutritional analyses performed by independent third-party laboratories and from data published by the USDA, respectively.

When the nutrient content of single servings of Green Magma was compared to the nutrient content of single servings of different vegetables, Green Magma was found to contain greater amounts of vitamin A, vitamins C, B$_1$, B$_2$, B$_3$, B$_6$, pantothenic acid, magnesium, and calcium than nine or more of the 10 vegetables measured. When compared to a 4.5-cup (>340-gram) salad of alfalfa sprouts, cabbage, celery, cucumber, lettuce, spinach, and tomato, Green Magma had five grams fewer carbohydrates but contained more vitamin A, vitamin C, vitamin B1, vitamin B$_6$, and pantothenic acid, and almost the same magnesium.

The above comparisons indicate that Green Magma provides comparable nutritional support to that of the recommended daily servings of fresh vegetables. Although only essential nutrients were measured, it can be inferred that the comparison also holds true for the diverse array of beneficial phytonutrients.

It is important to note that Green Magma is lower in carbohydrates than is the quantity of vegetables needed to provide the same amounts of essential nutrients as Green Magma. This is an important consideration for people on low-carbohydrate diets and for those concerned about their weight, since we know that body mass is directly linked to insulin resistance, which is linked to refined carbohydrate consumption.

Although one should not forgo vegetables for any supplement, taking a supplement that, together with a healthful diet, ensures that you receive both the quantity and diversity of needed phytonutrients can provide dramatic and long-lasting health benefits, including maximum health, vitality, and longevity.

In addition to barley grass, other green foods including broccoli, kale, cabbage, alfalfa, green tea, and spinach also contain concentrated amounts of certain phytonutrients with specific health benefits. In order to reap the benefits of these many different nutrients and phytonutrients from green foods and other nutritious vegetables without the hassle of juicing, Green Foods Corporation has developed a product called Veggie Magma®. This potent powdered vegetable combination is made with 18 vegetables and other botanicals, most of which have been juiced before being dried to a powder. Juicing releases the nutrients from the plant, thereby concentrating them and making them more bioavailable.

Veggie Magma's phytonutrients have broad-spectrum health benefits.

Green Magma: Free of Pesticides and Herbicides

I am a strong proponent of organic foods. Studies point to a variety of diseases that can be linked to pesticide and herbicide intake. When you buy food raised organically, you are not only protecting the health of yourself and your loved ones, you are also protecting the air, water, and soil, as well as animals from birds to bees and butterflies.

The Green Foods Corporation, along with other concerned companies in the natural food and supplement industries, supports and practices organic and sustainable farming methods. All the produce that Green Foods grows for use as ingredients in its products is certified organic. For all other ingredients that it purchases from other growers and raw-material vendors, Green Foods requires documentation of safety and purity. While many of these ingredients may not be available as organic due to practical, seasonal, and economic reasons, they are free of detectable levels of contaminants, including pesticide and herbicide residues.

Green Magma is not only free of detectable levels of pesticides and herbicides, its barley-grass-juice content may also help protect against pesticides in our diet from other sources.

The following is a description of Veggie Magma's ingredients and their known benefits.

Alfalfa: This contains nutrient-rich vitamins A, D, E, and K, phosphorous, iron, potassium, magnesium, and calcium. It is also rich in trace minerals, and its alkalinity helps the body assimilate proteins. It contains a group of compounds known as saponins, which lower blood cholesterol levels by combining with fats in the digestive tract, thereby helping the body to excrete them.

Aloe Vera contains calcium, potassium, sodium, manganese, iron, zinc, and lecithin. Aloe Vera also has 20 of 22 amino acids, including 10 essential amino acids.

Barley Grass: See box on page 43.

Broccoli contains sulforaphane, which may have antimutagenic properties. Broccoli is also a rich source of carotenoids, vitamin C, and folate.

Broccoli Sprouts have been found by scientists at Johns Hopkins University to contain 30 to 50 times more sulforaphane than mature broccoli.
Sulforaphane belongs to a class of phytonutrients known as isothiocyanates, which are known to strongly stimulate the induction of phase-2
enzymes, known to inactivate carcinogens.

Carrots are one the best sources of alpha- and beta-carotene, two lipid-
soluble antioxidants that inhibit free-radical formation and resulting inflammation. These two carotenoids also are used by the body to produce
vitamin A. Carrots contain moderate amounts of glutathione, a compound that helps recycle vitamin E and that has been shown to increase
the body's production of white blood cells. Carrots are also known to
strengthen the eyes.

Celery is plentiful in vitamins A and C, calcium, folic acid, and potassium.

Garlic contains allylic sulfides that may possess antimutagenic properties, enhance immune function, and offer cardiovascular protection. Allylic sulfides have also been found to inhibit fungal parasite growth and
reduce both cholesterol levels and blood platelet adhesion. As do cruci-
erous vegetables, garlic stimulates liver detoxification enzymes and helps
counteract microbial toxins.

Ginger root stimulates digestion and acts as an antioxidant preventing
lipid peroxidation.

Green Pepper contains vitamin C and has antimicrobial properties.

Kale contains sulforaphane and other isothiocyanates. It also contains a
rich variety of nutrients and phytonutrients—four times as much beta-

carotene as broccoli, more vitamin C than oranges, the highest concentration of lutein (a carotenoid antioxidant), and high amounts of antioxidant bioflavonoids, known to be important for cardiovascular health.

Red Beets are alkaline, contain high amounts of phosphorous and potassium, and stimulate digestion. They also contain betalains, water-soluble, reddish-purple pigments that, like the other three major types of pigments—chlorophyll, carotenoids, and flavonoids—possess antioxidant and detoxifying properties. Betalains stimulate the production of phase-2 enzymes that slow some risks of aging, including cancer and cardiovascular disease. Red beets also contain the amino acid betaine, which serves as a methyl donor. The donation of methyl groups by betaine is important for proper liver function, cellular replication, and detoxification reactions.

Shiitake Mushrooms contain the antimutagen polysaccharide lentinin, and have a high concentration of vitamin B complex, including vitamin B_{12} (a B vitamin that may be lacking in vegetarian diets). Other compounds in shiitake mushrooms may help lower cholesterol.

Spinach is high in blood-building iron, chlorophyll, folic acid, and beta-carotene, and has moderate amounts of the antioxidant glutathione.

Tomatoes are a rich source of lycopene, an antioxidant carotenoid. Tomatoes also contain high amounts of vitamin C, potassium, folic acid, beta-carotene, gamma-carotene, glutathione, and bioflavonoids.

I use both the powdered varieties of Green Magma and Veggie Magma, mixing 2 tablespoons in water. They are also great additions to smoothies.

GREEN TEA—AN IMPORTANT ALLY AGAINST AGE FORMATION

There has been a lot of speculation in recent years about green tea and its effects on insulin production. Despite its association with improved weight control, the record of green tea as a proven antidiabetes agent has been mixed at best, with clearly positive results reported from only one clinical trial, which tested the effects of a green tea extract.

But findings published in early 2007 by researchers from Swiss manufacturer DSM Nutritional Products show that green tea extract improves glucose tolerance in diabetic mice, an effect that could help prevent type 2 diabetes.

We should note at the outset that these encouraging results relate to DSM's highly concentrated green tea extract. The extract, called Teavigo™, contains unnaturally high levels (94% by weight) of one of tea's major polyphenol antioxidants, epigallocatechin gallate, or EGCG.

EGCG is believed to be responsible for much of green tea's promise in the prevention of cardiovascular disease, obesity, Alzheimer's disease, cancer, periodontal disease, and dental cavities. In addition, EGCG is "glucostatic." This simply means that EGCG helps prevent sharp rises in blood sugar and consequent spikes in insulin levels, key goals in the prevention and amelioration of diabetes, aging, metabolic disturbances, and the formation of AGEs.

The Swiss DSM team, led by Sven Wolfram, Ph.D., gave severely diabetic mice one of three different doses of EGCG or a placebo for seven weeks. They then administered glucose-tolerance tests after five weeks and insulin-tolerance tests after six weeks. They found that the animals' glucose tolerance improved after five weeks in a dose-dependent manner, with the effect being most noticeable in mice placed on a very-low-calorie diet.

Despite use of an EGCG-rich extract in the successful study, rather than the beverage itself, it seems reasonable to suppose that green tea offers real antidiabetes potential—another good reason to drink green tea or take a green tea extract frequently.

TURMERIC—THE SPICE FOR THE AGELESS

Turmeric is a member of the ginger family, and like ginger, it has long been used in India and China as a folk medicine, food preservative, coloring agent, and spice. Turmeric offers so many outstanding health benefits that it is almost in a class by itself. The deep-orange root of the turmeric plant contains a variety of polyphenol compounds called curcuminoids, which are close cousins to the polyphenol-class antioxidants that provide the cardiac and cancer-preventive properties in tea, chocolate, berries, ginger, grapes, plums, and other fruits, vegetables, herbs, and spices.

The oily substance called curcumin is the key to both turmeric's yellow-orange color and its health benefits. This is because curcumin consists of three particularly potent curcuminoid polyphenols called turmerone, atlantone, and zingiberone. Compared with the polyphenols in other plant foods, these curcuminoids possess extraordinarily strong antioxidant and anti-inflammatory properties. (Although it sounds similar, curcumin is not related to cumin, the popular seed used in chili and other Mexican and Spanish dishes.)

To date, curcumin has demonstrated the following key health properties. It:

- Interferes with all three stages of cancer formation: initiation, promotion, and progression;

- Reduces the inflammation, oxidation, and amyloid plaques associated with Alzheimer's disease;

- Acts as a powerful antioxidant and anti-inflammatory whose free radical–scavenging activity exceeds that of vitamin C and most polyphenols, including vitamin E and the catechins in tea and the flavonols in cocoa and dark chocolate;

- Exerts anti-inflammatory effects comparable to steroidal and non-steroidal drugs (e.g., aspirin, ibuprofen, naproxen);

- Protects the cardiovascular system by lowering triglyceride and cholesterol levels, reversing cell-membrane damage, and inhibiting inflammation and platelet aggregation;

- Protects the liver by several mechanisms;

- Ameliorates brain damage resulting from head trauma; and

- Enhances therapeutic benefits when used in conjunction with cold-water fish or omega-3 fish oil.

While curcumin constitutes only 3 to 5% of turmeric, a little bit packs a big preventive health punch, as you will see.

Age Less with More Turmeric

As we have learned, AGEs are compounds that form from the breakdown of sugars in the body. AGEs form constantly and slowly in the human body, and accumulate over time. However, diabetics experience increased incidences of tissue damage because their high blood sugar levels expedite the chemical reactions that form AGEs.

To explore the relationship among AGEs, diabetes, and curcumin, researchers administered oral does of curcumin to diabetic rats over a period of eight weeks. The rats received 200 milligrams of curcumin for every kilogram of body weight per day.

After the upsurge in curcumin consumption, the researchers examined the levels of antioxidants and AGEs, in addition to the rats' skin. They found that the rats' consumption of curcumin significantly reduced their oxidative stress.

This is important because we know that AGEs build up at a faster rate in the body when blood-sugar levels are elevated, as in diabetes. However, as we now know, and as this book points out, the elevated blood-sugar and insulin levels of nondiabetic children and adults in today's society are headed off the charts. To prevent these degenerative conditions, we need to implement many of the health and dietary strategies recommended for diabetics. Using turmeric liberally in a variety of recipes, and taking turmeric supplements as a proven preventative, may help slow the process of aging and promote youthfulness in all organ systems—including the skin.

Turmeric, Not Aspirin

Diabetes isn't the only area in which turmeric is proving helpful. Many exciting studies are showing how powerful it is in the prevention of Alzheimer's disease (AD) and other forms of dementia (remember that AGEs are found in significant quantities in the brains of

Alzheimer's patients). The curcumin in turmeric has also been shown to help immune-system cells clear damaging plaques from the brains of Alzheimer's patients (more about this later). This discovery was prompted by the realization that people from and in India enjoy substantially lower rates of AD than people from the U.S. and Europe. Since diet plays such a major role in health and disease, a search for dietary factors was undertaken to explain this enormous advantage. It didn't take long for researchers to discover that curry, a dish widely consumed in India, held the key, thanks to turmeric (an important curry component) and its family of powerful anti-AGEing chemicals, including curcumin.

Inflammation is both a promoter of and an effect of AD, which is why regular use of nonsteroidal anti-inflammatory drugs (NSAIDs) such as aspirin and ibuprofen seems to reduce the risk of developing Alzheimer's disease and reduce its severity and progression. Aspirin and other NSAIDs inhibit inflammation by blocking a multipurpose enzyme called cyclooxygenase-1 (COX-1), which can play a pro-inflammatory role. However, chronic use of NSAIDs can also cause gastrointestinal, liver, and kidney damage.

Thanks to earlier animal and human research on arthritis, scientists already knew that curcumin had strong antioxidant and anti-inflammatory properties, including the ability to block the activation of another pro-inflammatory enzyme, COX-2. However, unlike synthetic COX-2–inhibiting NSAIDs such as Vioxx and Celebrex, curcumin blocks the COX-2 enzyme without producing adverse cardiovascular effects. As the authors of a recent evidence review said, curcumin is "... a pharmacologically safe phytochemical agent ..." that inhibits excessive activation of pro-inflammatory genetic switches like nuclear factor kappa B (Nf-κB), which promote premature aging, AD, and cancer.

Need to Find Your Keys? Look for Turmeric

Epidemiological (population) studies looking for links between diet and health suggest that lovers of turmeric-rich curries cut their risk of senility by about 50%, while even occasional enjoyment of curry reduces dementia risk by 38%. AD is characterized by the formation of plaques made of inflammation-inducing proteins called beta-amyloids, which also form wiry tangles called fibrils.

No one is yet certain whether beta-amyloid plaques and fibrils cause or result from the still-mysterious process that leads to AD. But it *is* certain that beta-amyloid plaques and fibrils accompany AD symptoms, and that drugs and dietary factors that inhibit inflammation, oxidation, and formation of beta-amyloid plaques and fibrils also reduce AD symptoms.

It is the job of macrophages, special immune-system cells in our blood, to remove the beta-amyloid from our brains. Unfortunately, for many people these macrophages don't function properly. This weakens our immune system and also places us at greater risk for the brain-damaging inflammation characteristic of AD.

According to researchers at the University of California Los Angeles (UCLA) School of Medicine, curcumin enhances the ability of macrophages to remove plaques from brain tissues taken from AD patients. This study, conducted with AD patients and healthy controls, exposed macrophages to turmeric extract for 24 hours. The outcome of the study was very exciting. The turmeric-treated macrophages were able to function properly, removing the beta-amyloid plaques from the brain tissues. These initial findings may lead to an entirely new approach in treating AD. I am particularly enthusiastic about findings such as these because they demonstrate that enhancing the natural function of the immune system with natural substances can not only increase the body's ability to remove plaques that may cause AD and other forms of dementia, it also does so safely, effectively, and with no side effects.

Turmeric—The Smart Spice

The good news doesn't stop with AD. Turmeric has also been shown to enhance general cognitive performance. It's not a stretch to say that it appears to actually make people more adept at many mental tasks—including finding one's car keys. Researchers at the National University of Singapore recruited 1,010 older Asians (average age 68.9), questioned them about their curry intake, and placed them into one of three curry-consumption categories:

- "often or very often" (once a month to daily; 43% of participants)

- "occasionally" (41% of participants)

- "rarely or never" (16% of participants).

Lead researcher Tze-Pin Ng, M.D. Ph.D., and his colleagues then administered a standard brain function test called the Mini-Mental State Examination (MMSE), and compared the participants' test performances with their curry consumption.

It turned out that those who consumed curry "often or very often" were 49% less likely to display cognitive impairment, compared to those who rarely or never consumed it, while eating curry "occasionally" was associated with a 38% lower risk.

"These findings present the first epidemiological evidence supporting a link between curry consumption and cognitive performance that was suggested by a large number [sic] of earlier experimental evidence," Dr. Ng stated.

The study did have limitations, since it didn't take into account other possible risk-reducing or risk-promoting factors in the curry dishes, such as vegetables and fats, and the accuracy of self-reported curry consumption is not certain. Despite these limitations, the researchers point to turmeric as an obvious explanation for the observed differences between curry lovers and those who rarely consume it.

As Dr. Ng noted, "Interestingly, it has also been purported that the prevalence of Alzheimer's disease in India among the elderly between 70 and 79 years of age is fourfold less than that of the United States. The results reported here are therefore significant, as they point to a significant beneficial effect on cognitive functioning with even low to moderate levels of curry consumption."

A One-Two Punch: Turmeric and DHA

The news about turmeric just gets better, as it turns out that its effects are enhanced by other substances such as DHA, one of the two main omega-3 fatty acids in cold-water fish that are high in healthy fat. In a study conducted at the Veterans' Research, Education and Clinical Center in Sepul-

Curry Facts

Pure unadulterated turmeric powder and the fresh root, available in most grocery stores and natural food stores, are the best sources of this important spice. However, most people get their turmeric intake from curry and curry powder. The English word curry—which encompasses all Indian spice mixtures—comes from the Tamil (South Indian) word "kari," meaning soup or sauce. Be aware that commercial curry powders are not reliable sources of turmeric. Look for a good organic curry powder that lists turmeric as the first or second ingredient. If you have access to an Indian market you should also be able to find turmeric-rich blends of curry powder. Otherwise, shop in a natural foods store like Whole Foods, Wild Oats, Trader Joe's, or your local co-op. These stores stock the best-quality brands of curry powder. You can also shop online. A good organic curry powder by Morton and Bassett can be found at worldpantry.com. Watch out for commercially prepared curry sauces, which can also contain high levels of omega-6 fats from soy, corn, and conventional sunflower or safflower oils, making them much less beneficial. Recipes containing turmeric or turmeric-rich curry powder blends will be more beneficial if they use oils that do not contain these AGE-producing fatty acids. Opt instead for extra-virgin olive oil, macadamia nut oil, grapeseed oil, or high-lignan flaxseed oil. Look for cold-pressed, organic varieties, purchase them in small batches, and store them in a dark, cool place. Flaxseed oil should be stored in the refrigerator.

Although curry recipes vary widely from region to region and country to country, just about all of them include turmeric. When I make curry dishes, I usually increase the amounts of many of the spices, including turmeric. This boosts both the flavor and the antioxidant profile of the dish. However, be careful and adjust to taste, as some of the ingredients in a good curry powder are hot, such as cayenne (red) pepper, and turmeric itself also packs some heat.

veda, California, researchers found that while NSAIDs could reduce accumulation of beta-amyloid plaques, they suppressed few inflammatory markers and did not reduce oxidative damage (in addition to presenting the safety concerns mentioned on page 51).

The Veteran's study researchers tested the combined effects of curcumin-rich turmeric and DHA in mice and found the combination highly effective. As they said, DHA "also limited amyloid, oxidative damage and synaptic and cognitive deficits in . . . [mice]. Both DHA and turmeric have favorable safety profiles, epidemiology [population study results] and efficacy, and may exert general anti-aging benefits (anti-cancer and cardioprotective)."

All of this research is very encouraging. Scientists have been searching for a drug that can help slow the accumulation of these beta-amyloid plaques. It is heartening to know that a delightful culinary spice may hold the key.

Joint Protection

AGEs can wreak havoc in many ways. They have even been found in the serum and synovial fluid of patients with rheumatoid arthritis—a disease in which the body's immune system attacks joints, causing hot, painful swelling and deformity. It's long been known that the curcumin fraction of turmeric can alleviate the symptoms of arthritis in animals, and it has also displayed strong therapeutic benefit to humans in preliminary clinical trials.

Back in 1980 scientists in India tested curcumin in 49 patients with rheumatoid arthritis. Half were given 1,200 mg of curcumin per day, and the rest received a standard dose of phenylbutazone, a strong synthetic NSAID. At the end of six weeks, both groups enjoyed similar improvement in morning stiffness and physical endurance.

In another Indian study the anti-inflammatory potency of curcumin was also tested in hospital patients who had either undergone surgery or suffered some kind of physical trauma. One third received curcumin (1,200 mg/day), one third received a placebo, and one third took phenylbutazone (300 mg/day), for three to five days. Curcumin was judged to be as effective as phenylbutazone.

And an animal study funded by the U.S. National Institutes of Health, and conducted at the University of Arizona in Tucson, demonstrated that a 41% curcuminoid extract had positive impact when tested on arthritic mice. This study found that:

- destruction of cartilage in the tibia was reduced by 66%, compared to the animals treated with a placebo solution.

- loss of bone mineral density (BMD) in the animals' thighs was reduced by 57%, compared to those that got the placebo solution.

The equivalent effective dose in humans would be just ¼ to ½ teaspoon of curcumin per day.

Turmeric extracts inhibited NF-κB, the nuclear transcription factor (genetic switch) that promotes inflammation via several pathways, including activation of the pro-inflammatory COX-enzyme. This makes turmeric an important ally not just for arthritis sufferers, but also for treating a host of inflammatory and AGE-related diseases, including asthma (increased AGEs are found in asthma patients), multiple sclerosis (which is exacerbated by the receptor for AGEs, known as RAGE), and inflammatory bowel disease (IBD) (RAGE is elevated in colon tissue samples).

Turmeric Takes on Cancer

Turmeric is also known for its anticancer properties. When we incorporate turmeric into our diet, we can begin to reap the benefits of Hippocrates's wisdom, seen in his statement approximately 2,500 years ago: "Let food be thy medicine and medicine be thy food."

As reliable data on cancer rates in India became available in the early 1990s, researchers found it curious that people's risk of leukemia and colon, breast, prostate, and lung cancer in that curry-loving country was 10 to 20 times lower than in the U.S. The correlation between Indians' plentiful curry consumption and radically lower rates of the cancers that are most common in the U.S. prompted researchers in both countries to begin testing curry spices for their anticancer potential. Not surprisingly, they found that curcumin is the leading anticancer compound in curry.

Much of the research into curcumin's powerful anticancer properties has been conducted at the University of Texas M.D. Anderson Cancer Center, one of the world's leading cancer-research labs. A scientific review published in 2005 by the Anderson team found that the efficacy, pharmacologic safety, and cost-effectiveness of curcuminoids encourage us to "get back to our roots."

I find this observation valid on two fronts. First, much ancient medicine and wisdom is still viable and important today. And second, the remarkable healing and disease-prevention abilities of roots such as turmeric show the importance of food as medicine and medicine as food. The confidence with which these researchers describe the anticancer value of curcumin—and of 6-gingerol, a curcumin-like component of ginger root—reflects the strength and abundance of the evidence that they found, cited below from their study:

- "The use of turmeric . . . for treatment of different inflammatory diseases has been described in Ayurveda and in traditional Chinese medicine for thousands of years. The active component of turmeric responsible for this activity, curcumin, was identified almost two centuries ago.

- "Because it can modulate the expression of several important molecular targets, curcumin is now being used to treat cancer, arthritis, diabetes, Crohn's disease, cardiovascular diseases, osteoporosis, Alzheimer's disease, psoriasis, and other pathologies.

- "Interestingly, 6-gingerol, a natural analog of curcumin derived from the root of ginger (Zingiber officinalis), exhibits a biologic activity profile similar to that of curcumin. Another example of how these root spices offer so many therapeutic benefits—and a good reason to add freshly grated ginger root to your meals."

The Anderson team is now conducting two human clinical trials, testing the ability of daily capsules of curcumin powder to retard growth of pancreatic and multiple myeloma cancers. Another trial is planned for patients with breast cancer.

The Anderson Cancer Center's patient encyclopedia entry on turmeric states: "A lipid base of lecithin, fish oils or essential fatty acids may also be used to enhance absorption." As with many nutrients and nutritional supplements, omega-3 fish oil capsules work synergistically to increase turmeric's benefits.

Finally, it appears that a little turmeric may go a long way. In a cell test whose results showed that curcumin inhibits skin cancer (melanoma), an Anderson Center team found that it was effective *regardless* of the amount used. They reported that "the [inflammatory, cancer-promoting] NF-κB machinery is suppressed by both short exposures to high concentrations of curcumin as well as by longer exposure to lower concentrations of curcumin." In other words, you don't have to take megadoses to gain the benefits. Just ¼ to ½ teaspoon added to soups, stews, stir-fries, and curries on a regular basis will confer the benefits.

CINNAMON—THE AGE REDUCER

Cinnamon's history as a spice and medicine dates back to ancient Egypt, and it is mentioned in the Bible. This aromatic tree bark also became one of the first commodities traded between the Near East and Europe. "Ceylon" (the former name of Sri Lanka) cinnamon, now grown around the world, is the best variety. Here are just a few of the reasons cinnamon is so effective in fighting against AGEs:

■ Cinnamon stimulates insulin receptors, and inhibits an enzyme that inactivates them, thereby increasing cells' ability to use glucose. Thus, cinnamon may significantly help people with adult-onset diabetes normalize their blood sugar levels. In fact, less than half a teaspoon per day of cinnamon reduces blood sugar levels in persons with adult-onset diabetes. Just one gram per day (approximately ¼ to ½ teaspoon) yields a 20% drop in blood sugar, and reduces cholesterol 7–27% and triglyceride levels 23–30% as well. This is tremendously important information for Perricone followers, as one of the keys to stopping the signs of aging on the face and body is the regulation of blood sugar. It appears that just swizzling a stick of cinnamon in your tea will provide blood sugar–lowering benefits.

- Cinnamon reduces AGEs in two ways: by inhibiting the release of an inflammatory fatty acid called arachidonic acid from platelet membranes, and by reducing production of an inflammatory prostaglandin (messenger) called thromboxane A2. These actions help reduce the tendency of blood platelets to clump together and reduce blood flow.

- Cinnamon's essential oils help stop the growth of bacteria and fungi. They even inhibit strains of the infectious yeast *Candida albicans* that are resistant to the common antifungal medication fluconazole.

- In a test comparing cinnamon with anise, ginger, licorice, mint, nutmeg, vanilla, and the synthetic food preservatives BHA and BHT, cinnamon prevented oxidation more effectively than anything but mint.

- The mere scent of cinnamon enhances the brain's cognitive processing, including attention, memory, and visual–motor speed.

- Cinnamon is prized in ayurvedic and Traditional Chinese Medicine for its warming qualities, and is used to provide relief from colds or flu. When you feel an infection coming on, try a tea of cinnamon bark and fresh ginger.

As you can see, there any many wonderful dietary solutions for counteracting AGEs. In addition, many foods and spices are rife with other healthful benefits, helping delay and/or prevent the unwanted signs of AGEs and aging.

4

The Guide to Anti-AGEs Shopping, Cooking, and Preparation

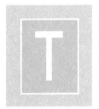 he purpose of this chapter is to show how to recognize and avoid the foods and methods of food preparation that trigger AGEs. I introduce non–AGE producing cooking methods that fight the aging of our skin and internal organs without sacrificing flavor.

As you have learned, certain foods, especially processed foods, contain AGEs as additives to influence their color and flavor. You have also learned that certain methods of food preparation promote the formation of AGEs. Foods cooked at high heat, for example, not only encourage the formation of these glycotoxins, they also promote the formation of cancer-causing toxins that mutate genes.

AGEs are also formed internally when we eat certain foods, such as sugars and starches. Sugar molecules bind to the RAGE, the receptor for AGE, resulting in increased inflammation and oxidative stress. This leads to many chronic and inflammatory diseases, including atherosclerosis, diabetes mellitus, kidney disease, AD, and other neurodegenerative diseases—as well as wrinkled, sagging skin. Fortunately, a lot of AGE formation is preventable, and it starts with the foods we eat and the methods we use to prepare them.

Remember, diet-derived AGEs that are absorbed into the bloodstream may represent a major source of toxins that are both chemically and biologically active. Because they are only partially eliminated in the urine, it stands to reason that those that remain in the body can have serious negative consequences. Help is at hand. You can greatly reduce the formation and storage of AGEs by learning which foods and preparation methods will block or significantly lessen their buildup in your body.

Let's start with the basics—the food we buy.

NAVIGATING THE SUPERMARKET

Wondering what to put in your cart? Use this guide for the healthiest and best-tasting food choices. When possible, shop at Wild Oats Markets, Whole Foods Markets, other natural food stores, co-ops, or the natural and organic section of your supermarket. That way you can be assured of the freshest foods as well as a wide choice of natural, organic, and unprocessed foods. With the exception of food high in saturated fats, such as grain-fed red meat, most fresh, unprocessed foods have the least potential to generate AGEs—a fact I remind you of throughout this book. I have also included some brand recommendations to help you make the best food choices and safely avoid undesirable ingredients. If you don't have access to stores such as those listed above, you can shop online. See the Resources section for many outstanding websites that will deliver the freshest salmon, organic fruits and vegetables, nuts and seeds, grass-fed beef, recommended cheeses, sheep and goat milk yogurt, and more.

Food Allergies

According to the excellent website of the Food Allergy & Anaphylaxis Network (FAAN), www.foodallergy.org, a food allergy is an immune-system response to a food that the body mistakenly believes is harmful. Once the immune system decides that a particular food is harmful, it creates specific antibodies to it. The next time that food is eaten, the immune system releases massive amounts of chemicals, including histamine, to protect the body from the threat. These chemicals trigger a cascade of allergic symptoms that can affect the respiratory system, gastrointestinal tract, skin, and cardiovascular system. Scientists estimate that approximately 12 million Americans suffer from true food allergies.

Although an individual can be allergic to any food, such as fruits, vegetables, and meats, there are eight foods that account for 90% of all food allergic reactions. These are milk, eggs, peanuts, tree nuts (such as walnuts, cashews), fish, shellfish, soy, and wheat.

About one person in 133 has an allergy to gluten, a substance found in wheat and other grains. Over the years, I have observed in my own medical practice that many of my patients have had a very low-grade or subclinical wheat or gluten allergy. This is manifested as a slight increase in subclinical inflammation and complaints of fatigue.

FAAN's "Do You Have a Food Allergy?" brochure, distributed at health fairs throughout the country, is available thanks to a grant from the American College of Allergy, Asthma & Immunology (ACAAI). You can download a copy from their website (www.foodallergy.org).

RECOMMENDED PROTEIN SOURCES

The proteins outlined below, cooked properly, are my recommendations for AGEless healthy aging.

Going Green in the Deep Blue

The Monterey Bay Aquarium is very helpful in compiling lists of seafood that are the best choices from an environmental as well as a health perspective. You will see in the following list that a number of different types of farmed seafood are recommended. Often we recommend wild seafood, but with every rule there are exceptions, and these are duly noted when the farming methods are efficient and safe for both the seafood and the environment. In other cases, a particular type of wild fish or shellfish will not be recommended because it has been overfished in its natural environment—often to the point of extinction. Also included are geographical recommendations, that is, which area has the recommended form of seafood—Alaskan versus Atlantic salmon, for example. If there is no recommendation or comment next to the seafood, all available forms are acceptable for consumption.

Best Sources of Omega-3 Seafood

These fatty, cold-water fish are the ideal protein source. Salmon, for example, is not only rich in heart-healthy omega-3s, it also contains a powerful carotenoid known as astaxanthin that helps counteract the damage from AGE-mediated inflammation.

Abbreviations used in the list below: AK, Alaska; BC, British Columbia; CA, California; OR, Oregon; U.S., United States; WA, Washington.

Wild Alaskan salmon, (CA, AK, wild-caught). Sockeye salmon has the highest amount of omega-3 of any fish, about 2.7 grams per 100-gram portion.

Anchovies	Sablefish/Black Cod, (AK, BC)
Halibut (Pacific)	Salmon (canned)
Herring	Sardines
Mackerel	Trout, rainbow (farmed)

Additional Seafood Recommendations

Abalone (farmed)	Oysters, farmed
Catfish (U.S., farmed)	Sea bass, white
Caviar (farmed)	Shrimp, prawns, (trap-caught)
Clams (farmed)	Squid (CA market squid)
Crab, Dungeness	Striped bass (farmed)
Halibut, Pacific	Sturgeon (farmed)
Lobster, Rock/Spiny (CA, Australia)	Tilapia (farmed)

Seafood that Comes with a Warning

There are some problems with the way these forms of seafood are either caught or farmed. However, these are better choices than the seafood that appears on the "seafood-to-avoid" list.

Clams (wild-caught)

Cod (Pacific)

Crab, Imitation/Surimi

Crab, king (AK)

Crab, snow

Sablefish/black Cod (CA, WA, OR)

Salmon (OR, WA wild-caught)

Sand dabs, Pacific

Scallops, bay, sea

Shark, thresher, (U.S., West coast)

Shrimp (U.S., farmed or wild-caught)

Sole, English/Dover/petrale Rex

Lobster, American

Mahi mahi

Mussels (wild-caught)

Oysters (wild-caught)

Pollock

Swordfish (U.S. West coast)

Tuna, albacore/bigeye/yellowfin (longline or purse seine–caught)

Tuna, canned

Seafood to Avoid

These fish come from sources that are overfished, or they are caught or farmed in ways that harm the environment.

Caviar, beluga/osetra/sevruga

Chilean sea bass

Cod, Atlantic/Icelandic

Crab, king (imported)

Lingcod

Monkfish

Orange roughy

Rockfish/rock cod/Pacific snapper

Salmon (farmed/Atlantic)

Sharks (except U.S. West coast thresher)

Shrimp (imported)

Sturgeon (wild-caught)

Swordfish (Atlantic)

Tuna, bluefin

A Special Note on Seafood from the Environmental Protection Agency (EPA)

By following these two recommendations for selecting and eating fish or shellfish, women and young children will receive the benefits of these foods while being confident that they have reduced their exposure to the harmful effects of mercury.

1. Do not eat shark, swordfish, king mackerel, or tilefish, because they contain high levels of mercury.

2. Eat up to 12 ounces (two average meals) a week of a variety of fish and shellfish that are lower in mercury.

- Five of the most commonly eaten fish that are low in mercury are shrimp, canned light tuna, salmon, pollock, and catfish.

- Another commonly eaten fish, albacore ("white") tuna has more mercury than canned light tuna. So, when choosing your two meals of fish and shellfish, you may eat up to six ounces (one average meal) of albacore tuna per week.

WHEN IT COMES TO POULTRY: SAFETY FIRST

As on any perishable meat, bacteria can be found on raw or undercooked chicken. They multiply rapidly at temperatures between 40° F and 140° F (out of refrigeration and before thorough cooking occurs). Freezing doesn't kill bacteria, but they are destroyed by thorough cooking.

Bacteria on food must be consumed to cause illness. They cannot enter the body through a skin cut. However, raw poultry must be handled carefully to prevent cross-contamination. This can occur if raw poultry or its juices contact cooked food or foods that will be eaten raw such as salad. An example of this is chopping tomatoes on an unwashed cutting board just after cutting raw chicken on it. Always wash and dry your hands, cutting boards, knives, and other utensils thoroughly when handling raw poultry to prevent any cross-contamination. I also recommend that you use two cutting boards—one exclusively for meat, the other one for fruits and vegetables.

A Cutting Board for a Green Planet

When it comes to choosing a sustainable and durable cutting board, I recommend that you choose one made from bamboo. Bamboo is a grass, not a tree, and it can grow as much as two feet or more in one day. There is no need to replant bamboo once it is harvested, because it will grow a new shoot from its extensive root system. Unlike hardwood trees, which are gone forever once they are cut down, bamboo continuously renews itself, providing us with an endlessly renewable resource.

Best Poultry Choices

Organic, free-range chicken and turkey

Cornish hens

Turkey sausage and bacon (avoid any products with nitrates; see Chapter Two for information on the dangers of nitrates).

When possible, look for free-range poultry that has not been given antibiotics and/or growth hormones. Additives are not permitted on fresh chicken. If chicken is processed, however, additives such as MSG, salt, or sodium erythorbate—additives that you should avoid—may be added but must be listed on the label.

Recommended poultry brands include Coleman's and Organic Valley. Diamond Organics also has a great selection of organic Kosher poultry available at *www.diamondorganics.com.* Whole Foods and Wild Oats Markets also provide a large selection of organic, free-range poultry.

When shopping for poultry, look for these qualities:

▪ Produced without pesticides, antibiotics, or hormones

▪ 100% certified organic feed

▪ Humane treatment of animals

▪ Family farmer produced

- Poultry is free ranging, with full access to the outdoors

- No animal by-products used in feed

- No nitrates, nitrites, or preservatives

THE EGG QUESTION

In the past there has been much discussion about the cholesterol content of eggs. Research indicates that when eggs are eaten as part of a low-fat diet, they are unlikely to alter blood lipid levels (cholesterol). Of much greater importance is the risk posed by a family history of heart disease and a high intake of saturated and trans fats. However, if you have a cholesterol problem, consult with your physician as to the recommended intake of eggs.

If you do choose to eat eggs, it is important to know what the chickens that laid them had for dinner. Chickens should be cage free and free range so that they can roam the barnyard eating the grasses, seeds, and insects that occur naturally. Any grains that they are fed should be organic, meaning that the chickens are fed foods that are pesticide free. Also make sure that the chickens have not been fed growth hormones or given antibiotics. Their diet should include foods such as organic flax to increase the omega-3 content of the eggs.

Although at one time a low-fat, high-carbohydrate diet was believed to be key in preventing insulin resistance, the available evidence now suggests otherwise. In its place, a diet with unsaturated fats such as those found in fish and high-fiber, low-glycemic carbohydrates, including low-fat, unsweetened dairy products, is our best bet. These foods will not disturb blood sugar and insulin, and will not boost the development of glycation or AGEs. So instead of that bagel for breakfast, reach for plain yogurt with some fresh fruit.

GET MILK?

These days, shoppers are confronted with a myriad of milk, cheese, and yogurt selections. Which are best for you? Nonorganic milk and dairy products can have residues of growth hormones and antibiotics. Added sugars and fruits may threaten the survival of the cultures that make yogurt and other cultured dairy foods like kefir and acidophilus milk, which are much healthier choices than plain milk products. Fresh fruit, nuts, seeds, and a sprinkle of cinnamon are healthy and tasty alternatives to presweetened yogurt. In general, watch your diary intake. Choose low-fat varieties of dairy from cow's milk. Sheep and goat yogurts and cheeses present a healthier profile than cow's milk varieties.

Best Dairy Products

Plain low-fat kefir

Plain low-fat yogurt

Buttermilk

Low-fat cottage cheese

Farmer's cheese

Low-fat ricotta cheese

When shopping for dairy products, follow these guidelines:

- Buy organic foods that are free of antibiotics, pesticides, and growth hormones.
- Read labels and avoid dairy products that contain the following ingredients:
  - sweeteners
  - potassium sorbate
  - fillers
  - stabilizers
  - guar gum
  - carageenan
  - food coloring.

Join the Culture Club

Many people are lactose intolerant, which means that they lack the ability to digest or absorb lactose, a type of sugar found in cow's milk and other dairy products. Lactose intolerance is caused by a deficiency of the enzyme lactase. Most people who are allergic to cow's milk or are lactose intolerant find that they can tolerate dairy products made from goat and sheep milk. This is especially true when it comes to yogurt, because yogurt cultures convert lactose into lactic acid, making yogurt easier to digest than milk. The yogurt cultures lactobacillus, acidophilus, and bifidus can also help restore normal intestinal flora after antibiotic therapy. Because yogurt is easier to digest than milk, people who cannot drink cow's milk often find that they can eat yogurt made from cow's milk. However, because many people cannot even tolerate cow's milk yogurt, it is good to know that there are excellent alternatives, such as goat or sheep milk yogurt and cheese.

One delicious variety of yogurt that I enjoy is Redwood Hill Farm Goat Milk Yogurt (see Resource Section for purchasing information). Although it is not low fat, it has a much healthier fat than the fat in cow's milk. Goat milk's ease of digestibility is due to the fact that it has smaller fat particles than the ones found in cow's milk. It is also a good source of calcium, protein, phosphorous, vitamin B_{12}, and potassium.

Willow Hill Farm is a certified organic farm that offers internationally award-winning Vermont sheep and cow's milk cheeses and sheep yogurt. Thick, tangy, creamy, and rich, sheep milk has some very interesting characteristics that make it a natural for yogurt production. Sheep's milk

- has more of the vitamins A, B, C, and E than cow's milk

- has twice the calcium and higher levels of the minerals phosphorus, potassium, and magnesium than cow's milk

- has less sodium than cow's milk

- has more protein than cow's milk

- is easier to digest than cow's milk for some people, due to its inherently smaller fat particles

- is made up of short-chain fatty acids that have been found to have little effect on human cholesterol levels

- is gluten free. You might ask yourself, why would there be gluten in yogurt? There answer is that there may be trace amounts of gluten in yogurt that contains fruit from the processing of the fruit and flavors with a grain alcohol. This is another important reason to purchase plain yogurt and add your own fresh fruit

- has no trans fats. You might not expect yogurt to have trans fats either, but trans fats are produced naturally in the stomachs of cows; hence their presence in dairy products. Unlike industrial trans fats, they do not appear to cause heart disease. However, it seems like a good idea to avoid them if possible—and sheep's milk solves that problem

If separation occurs in your yogurt, just stir the liquid back into the yogurt. Greek-style yogurt such as the Fage brand is strained to remove liquid whey, resulting in a naturally thickened product with the consistency of sour cream.

Buttermilk

All commercially sold buttermilk is cultured. This means that a safe lactic acid–producing bacterial culture is added to freshly pasteurized skim or low-fat milk to produce the buttermilk. Buttermilk is much thicker than skim milk, and is higher in sodium than other milk. And buttermilk is a good thirst quencher.

Always keep cultured buttermilk chilled. If it is allowed to warm, it may separate. If it does separate, just stir it back together.

Say Cheese

Cheese is a delicious food that has been enjoyed worldwide for centuries. The good news about cheese for the lactose intolerant is that most cheeses have little or no lactose. The milk sugar is consumed in the fermentation

Fat Content of Cow's Milk Products

SELECTED PRODUCTS	TOTAL FAT GRAMS	SATURATED FATTY ACIDS GRAMS	CHOLESTEROL MILLIGRAMS
1 cup milk			
skim	trace	trace	4
1%	3	2	10
2%	5	3	18
whole	8	5	33
1 cup yogurt			
nonfat plain	trace	trace	4
low-fat plain	4	2	15
½ cup cottage cheese			
low-fat, 1% fat	1	1	5
creamed	5	3	16
1 oz. cheese			
mozzarella	5	3	15
natural cheddar	9	6	29

COURTESY USDA

and aging process, so *aged* cheeses should not present any problems. Cheeses like cottage cheese are not aged, so they have some lactose— about three grams per serving for cottage cheese, compared to 12 grams in an eight-ounce glass of milk.

Lactose intolerance aside, many cheeses are high in saturated fat, so it is best to enjoy them in moderation. A good way to do this is to purchase the oldest, sharpest varieties. You will find that cheddar cheese, for example, that is aged more than two years will taste much sharper. This will enable you to eat a smaller amount to satisfy your cheese craving. Pair it with a crisp apple for the ideal balance of taste and texture.

Cheese, like most dairy products, is a good source of protein, vitamins, minerals, fat, saturated fat, and cholesterol. Cheese is also an excellent source of calcium. According to the USDA, a 1½-ounce serving of natural cheese supplies the same amount of calcium as one cup of milk or yogurt, as well as 12 to 14 grams total fat, 9 grams saturated fat, 44 milligrams cholesterol, and 173 calories. For sodium, while one cup of milk contains 120 milligrams, 1½ ounces of natural cheese can contain from 110 to 450 milligrams, while two ounces of processed cheese can contain 800 milligrams. I strongly recommend that you avoid processed cheese products because, in addition to all the sodium, there can be many artificial colorings, flavorings, and so forth. In fact, much of the popular processed "cheese" products in your supermarket are not real cheese and actually contain no cheese at all. They are made from MPC (milk protein concentrate). You will notice that these "cheeses" do not use the word "cheese" on their labels, but rather modified versions of the word. I recommend avoiding them totally. Opt for real cheese.

When it comes to choosing cheese, the strong, aged cheeses such as the grating cheeses listed below have much more flavor than young cheeses. This helps us use less without sacrificing taste.

RECOMMENDED CHEESES:

Organic low-fat cottage cheese

Organic crumbly cheeses such as feta, especially feta from sheep or goat's milk

Farmer's cheese. These cheeses are much lower in saturated fats than cheeses that are solid at room temperature like cheddar, muenster, and Swiss.

Goat cheese, like goat milk, is easier on the human digestive system, and is lower in calories, cholesterol, and fat than its bovine counterpart. Goat cheese is rich in calcium, protein, vitamin A, vitamin K, phosphorus, niacin, and thiamine.

Part-skim mozzarella

Part-skim ricotta

Reduced fat Swiss or Jarlsberg

I recommend hard grating cheeses such as parmigiana Reggiano, an aged, imported cow's milk cheese, and pecorino Romano, which is made from a part-skim sheep's milk. Both of these cheeses will impart tremendous flavor to any dish, and a little goes a long way.

If you like to have cream cheese with your smoked salmon (just remember to skip the bagel), try substituting Neufchâtel. This French cheese has the same creamy consistency and mild taste but is lower in fat than its American cousin. When choosing cream cheese-type products, be sure to *read the label.* Many of them contain ingredients that you don't need, including stabilizers such as xanthan, carob bean, and guar gums, and preservatives such as sorbic acid. A good choice is Organic Valley cheeses. See the Resources section for purchasing information.

Here is a selection of popular higher-fat cheeses to enjoy in moderation:

Brie	Gruyère
Camembert	Jarlsberg
Cheddar	Muenster
Edam	Port du Salut
Fresh Mozzarella	Provolone
Gouda	Swiss

AGE-PREVENTION IN A NUTSHELL OR A SEED POD

Nuts and seeds should be organic, unsalted, and unroasted. Purchase your nuts and seeds in small quantities and store them in the refrigerator or freezer. Nuts and seeds make a delicious and nutritious alternative to bread crumbs when you want a coating for chicken, tofu, or seafood. You will find that your food has a delightful nutty flavor; it will also have additional nutrients, including essential healthy monounsaturated fats, phytonutrients, and protein.

Nut butters are nutritious but they are high in fat. Even though they contain healthy fat—providing that you are purchasing brands without hydrogenated vegetable oils—nut butters should be used in moderation to prevent unwanted weight gain because they are very calorie dense. They need to be kept refrigerated to prevent rancidity. For optimum freshness, you can make your own. Just add nuts or seeds to a small grinder such as those used for grinding coffee beans. Small batches will be used more rapidly than large jars of purchased nut butters, helping maintain freshness.

Healthy nut choices include:

Almonds	Pecans
Brazil nuts	Pine nuts (pignoli)
Butternuts (aka white walnuts)	Pistachios (white shell)
Flax seeds	Pumpkin and squash seeds
Hazelnuts (filberts)	Sesame seeds
Macadamia nuts	Sunflower seeds
Organic unsalted seeds	Walnuts

Almond Joy

Just as many foods wreak havoc with our blood-sugar and insulin levels (think pasta, bagels, and chips) and promote the formation of AGEs, other foods help stabilize blood sugar. These foods include almonds, one of my favorite nuts. Almonds are as versatile as they are delicious.

Interestingly many of the foods that promote AGE formation also increase the appetite, such as foods made with flour, sugar, and/or high-fructose corn syrup. Exciting new studies from Canada help explain how almonds curb the appetite.

A team at the University of Toronto reports that eating almonds can decrease our glycemic (blood-sugar) and insulin responses to high-carbohydrate meals (Jenkins, D.J. et al., 2006), the factors that increase appetite. This finding is very exciting, because if we decrease these responses, we will decrease both appetite and AGE formation.

As study coauthor Cyril Kendall said, "Almonds have already been found to reduce LDL [low-density lipoprotein] cholesterol levels and contain a variety of important nutrients. This new research shows that incorporating almonds in the diet may help in the management of blood glucose levels and the onset of such illnesses as diabetes, while promoting a healthy heart." Remember that AGE formation is directly related to high blood-glucose levels.

The researchers recruited 15 healthy volunteers (seven men, eight women) and tested the effects of five meals, eaten on five different occasions, on the levels of glucose, insulin, and antioxidants in their blood. The subjects ate two control meals that included bread, and three test meals that included: almonds and bread; parboiled rice; and instant mashed potatoes. All the meals had identical carbohydrate, fat, and protein content. Butter and cheese were used to adjust the proportions of each. The almonds-and-bread meal included 60 grams (two ounces) of almonds.

As expected, the glycemic indices (rises in blood sugar) following the rice meals and almonds-added meals were much lower than the indices following the potato meal: glycemic indices of 38 and 55 versus 94, respectively.

In the meals that contained the almonds, the researchers also noted that there was a reduction in the markers of free-radical damage in the volunteers' blood, most likely due to the very high antioxidant content of the almond skins.

As the authors wrote, "These actions may relate to mechanisms by which nuts are associated with a decreased risk of CHD [coronary heart disease]."

It isn't practical to consume two ounces (about a handful) of almonds with every high-carb meal, but that isn't the point. Instead, the purpose of the study was to see whether almonds are antiglycemic, and they certainly proved to be that. And as we have learned, antiglycemic is also anti-AGEs.

So add a few almonds to the dietary picture when you can. Besides being a bread-crumb substitute, you can add sliced or chopped almonds to green beans for the classic green beans amandine. I also add almonds to salads. You can also sprinkle them on cereal, salads, or yogurt, and enjoy them with an apple and a slice of cheese as a snack. Raw, organic almond butter is also a much healthier and better-tasting alternative to peanut butter.

FULL OF BEANS (AND LENTILS)

I start this section with the subhead "Full of Beans" because this delightful idiom means full of energy and enthusiasm, and that is how you will feel when you add these delicious legumes to your diet. Beans and lentils come in a great many shapes, sizes, colors, and varieties. It is heartening to see that even traditional supermarkets are now setting up aisles that contain dispensers filled with a vast selection of these nutrient powerhouses.

Beans and lentils are true superstars in the plant food kingdom. Incredibly inexpensive (even the organic varieties), beans and lentils provide excellent satiety—a soup, stew, or side dish made with this high-protein form of healthy carbohydrates will ensure that you will not leave the table hungry.

Required Eating

Beans and lentils offer many benefits in the prevention of AGE formation, starting with their ability to stabilize blood sugar. In fact, they have truly exceptional powers in this department, and should be required eating by everyone wanting to block AGEs and aging. Beans and lentils are also high in antioxidant phytonutrients that reduce AGE-mediated inflammation. Ounce for ounce, beans and lentils encourage the body to burn rather than store fat, all the while providing more protein than any other plant food.

Because elevated glucose and insulin are implicated in just about every disease or unhealthy condition, from obesity to AGEs, beans and lentils are an important strategic intervention. They not only ensure that blood sugar will rise very slowly and moderately after a meal, they will also work their magic at your next meal as well, moderating your blood-sugar response regardless of whether or not that meal includes beans or lentils.

Carb Insurance

For all of us who are guilty at times of eating foods higher on the glycemic index than we should, here is more good news. Even when they are eaten with relatively high-glycemic foods (sugars or refined flour products such as pasta or bread), beans and lentils still wield a potent stabilizing influence on blood-sugar levels and subsequent insulin levels. Because of this, I recommend that whenever you have a meal that includes pasta, for example, add beans such as chickpeas to the dish to moderate the glycemic effect. Also, add chickpeas or other varieties of beans (or lentils) to all of your soups, stews, and salads—this is a good habit to adopt, and a great way to increase your all-important fiber intake.

It is beans' and lentils' high level of nondigestible starch (known as fiber) that helps block AGE formation. Western diets are woefully deficient in fiber—a key reason we weigh more and have more body fat and higher body mass indexes than traditional native cultures whose diets are fiber rich and devoid of processed, refined foods.

An interesting article, published by the *New England Journal of Medicine* and reported by the Medical College of Wisconsin, found that diabetic patients who included 50 grams of fiber in their daily diet lowered their glucose levels by 10%. Fifty grams is a lot of fiber, about twice as much as the American Diabetes Association recommends, and nearly three times as much fiber as most Americans consume in a day. In addition, some researchers believe that if we eat 40 to 50 grams of fiber per day we may interfere with vitamin and nutrient absorption. However, if most of us simply doubled the amount of healthy, high-fiber plant foods we currently consume, we would probably notice a significant decrease in the negative effects of elevated blood sugar.

The high-fiber diet reported in *NEJM* also decreased insulin levels in the blood, and lowered blood-lipid concentrations in study patients with type 2 diabetes, the most prevalent type. I believe that simply including beans and lentils daily at either lunch or dinner could potentially accomplish a similar goal.

Resistant Starch

In addition to AGE-blocking fiber, the second way beans and lentils help block AGE formation is due to the fact that, as mentioned above, they contain a substance known as resistant starch (RS), which resists digestion and absorption as it passes through the small intestine (where most dietary starch gets digested). However, unlike a true fiber, some portion of dietary RS does eventually get digested. But it happens much too slowly to produce an inflammatory spike in blood-sugar levels. Clinical studies show that RS has the ability to actually improve long-term insulin sensitivity, due to its probiotic, fermentation-increasing effects in the digestive system. RS goes past the stomach and small intestine before settling in the colon. There, bacteria attack it just as they do a dietary fiber, producing butyrate—a short-chain fatty acid desirable for its cancer-preventing qualities.

Legumes contain substantially higher percentages of RS than do cereal grains, flours, and grain-based food products.

THE WHOLE TRUTH ABOUT WHOLE GRAINS

We hear a whole lot about the health benefits of whole grains. Unfortunately, many so-called "whole-grain" products are not much better than their refined counterparts. Take bread for example. Very few breads are true examples of whole-grain cooking. If they were, the loaves would be as dense as bricks. Instead most of them contain copious amounts of regular refined flour.

According to the World Grain Council, to qualify for the term "whole grain," the grain or the food made from them must contain all the essential parts, including the bran, germ, and endosperm, and naturally occurring nutrients of the entire grain seed. If the grain has been processed (e.g., cracked, crushed, rolled, extruded, and/or cooked), the food product should deliver approximately the same rich balance of nutrients that is found in the original grain seed.

Epidemiological studies have found that a diet rich in whole grains is protective against cancer, heart disease, diabetes, and obesity. However, the benefits are the greatest when we consume three servings of whole grains per day. Like beans and legumes, whole grains are rich in fiber, RS, and oligosaccharides, an important form of carbohydrate. Whole grains are also high in antioxidants and a whole host of phytochemicals that can prevent disease.

Whole grains are also important allies in the quest for foods that help prevent AGEs. Regular consumption of whole grains decreases the risk of developing type 2 diabetes because they have a direct and positive effect on both glucose and insulin.

Researchers use the glycemic index as a biomarker to determine the relationship among glucose insulin metabolism, and the intake of whole grains. Many factors influence the glycemic index of foods, including the fat content, the fiber content, the type of food, and how it is processed and/or cooked. As we know, highly processed, refined foods are rapidly digested, while foods such as whole grains are digested more slowly. Researchers have found that foods in which the original structure is preserved, such as whole grains, beans, and legumes, are important determinants in the glycemic response in diabetics. I have also found this to be true in nondiabetics. The more natural and whole our foods are, the better they are at preventing AGE formation and all of its related health threats.

The simple act of refining grains creates a pro-AGE food in place of an anti-AGE one. It is that simple. Finely ground flour, for example, accelerates insulin insensitivity, that is, it causes insulin to be released. Whole grains, on the other hand, increase insulin sensitivity. Many of you are used to cooking rice, especially brown rice, on a regular basis. Oats, barley, buckwheat, quinoa, millet, amaranth, or wild rice can be used in any recipe calling for brown rice. Oats in particular, which have one of the lowest glycemic indexes of all grains, are particularly adaptable.

A special note on whole grains and cancer. Researchers have found that the incidence of colon cancer is linked to higher levels of blood glucose and insulin and higher body weight. They have observed that the similarity of lifestyle and environmental risk factors for type 2 diabetes and colon cancer are significantly related.

Recommended Whole Grains

Although wheat is a whole grain, I do not include it in this list of recommended grains because of its high gluten content.

Oats

Barley

Quinoa

Buckwheat

Oats

Oats are a good source of manganese, magnesium, selenium, and iron, as well as calcium, zinc, and copper. Oats also contain small but significant quantities of several of the essential vitamins, particularly thiamine, folic acid, biotin, and pantothenic acid. In recent years oats have attracted a lot of attention as "the heart-healthy grain," thanks to their cholesterol-lowering beta-glucan fibers. Oats are good for cardiovascular health and are also of benefit in weight control. Old-fashioned whole oats have a delightful nutty flavor; a hearty breakfast of old-fashioned whole oats or oatmeal, topped with fresh fruit, chopped nuts or seeds, and plain yogurt, will help keep you going for hours.

Oats and AGEs

Thanks to the beta-glucan fiber in oats, they are able to exercise beneficial antiglycemic effects. The results of a controlled clinical trial published in 2002 showed that diabetics given oatmeal, oat bran, or foods fortified with beta-glucan registered far lower and slower rises in blood sugar compared with volunteers who consumed the equal amount in the form of white rice or bread. Like beans and lentils, oats are excellent collaborators in our goal to keep blood sugar and insulin from rising rapidly.

There are many forms of oats, and almost all of them are excellent; however, for optimum fiber, avoid instant oatmeal. When choosing oats, look for the following varieties:

1. Whole groats. These are oats that look like large grains of rice. They are oats in their most natural, unprocessed state. Whole oats make an excellent substitute for rice, and can be cooked in the same manner, lending themselves to every conceivable type of dish from risotto to soups, chowders, stir-fries, and stews.

2. Steel-cut oats. These are 100% whole-grain oat groats that, rather than being rolled, have been cut into smaller pieces but are otherwise

unprocessed, for a full, hearty texture and rich, nutty taste. Cook as you would whole oats. They can be used as a breakfast cereal or as a replacement for less-desirable grains such as bulgur due to high gluten content.

3. Old-fashioned oatmeal, which is simply whole oat groats that have been rolled or flattened. All nutrients are intact; the rolling just enables them to cook more quickly. Oatmeal or rolled oats make an excellent breakfast cereal, and are also a delicious addition to soups and chowders.

Barley

Barley is a delicious, nutty, chewy grain as well as a staple food of the ancient world. Most people are familiar with pearl barley, a popular ingredient in soups. However, I recommend hulled barley. This is barley in its most unprocessed and nutritious form, rich in fiber, lignans, antioxidants, and a whole host of disease-preventing phytonutrients. Hulled barley, in which the outer hull (the bran) is left intact, is the only form of barley that can truly be called "whole grain," and is therefore the only form of barley useful in AGE prevention.

Barley is low glycemic and high in both *soluble* and *insoluble fiber.*

- Soluble fiber helps the body metabolize fats, cholesterol, and carbohydrates, and lowers blood-cholesterol levels.

- Insoluble fiber—commonly called "roughage"—promotes a healthy digestive tract and reduces the risk of cancers affecting it (e.g., colon cancer).

Fiber-rich barley is a powerful ally in the prevention of AGE formation because it slows the digestion of starch, helping keep blood-sugar levels stable. Barley, as well as the other whole grains, is also a rich source of lignans, phytonutrients that act as antioxidants. Lignans also help prevent many cancers, including breast cancer. Barley's high fiber content also helps speed food through the digestive tract, and because it's a good source of selenium, it has been shown to significantly reduce the risk of colon cancer.

Quinoa

Organic quinoa, pronounced "keen-wah" (*Chenopodium quinoa Willd*) is an ancient staple grain with great flavor and superior nourishment. And unlike other grains, it has the benefit of being extremely quick cooking. For close to three decades, Eden Organics has worked closely with a group of Ecuadorian farmers to produce the highest standard of organic quinoa, grown on small family plots at over 11,000 feet in the Andes mountains.

Quinoa is a gluten-free whole grain that can be tolerated by most people with allergies to grains. The American Celiac Sprue Association lists quinoa as "consistent with a gluten-free diet at this time. Versatile, it can be substituted for any grain, used whole as a hot cereal or ground into flour."

Quinoa has the best amino acid profile of all grains, including all the essential amino acids, and provides the most complete protein. It is also an excellent source of dietary fiber (45% per serving) and phosphorus, and is a good source of iron, vitamin E, riboflavin (vitamin B_2), vitamin B_6, magnesium, and zinc. It is naturally very low in sodium, and is saturated fat and cholesterol free.

Quinoa, like the other whole grains mentioned in this chapter, helps in AGE prevention because it slows the conversion of complex carbohydrates into sugar, thus helping maintain stable blood glucose and insulin levels.

Buckwheat

China, Japan, and Korea have cultivated buckwheat for at least 1,000 years. In Japan, buckwheat is enjoyed in the form of "soba" noodles. Although we have classified buckwheat as a whole grain, it is really a seed related to the rhubarb family. When people in the U.S. think of buckwheat, they often think of buckwheat pancakes. But buckwheat can also be used in cooking in the same ways as other whole grains. Buckwheat also ranks low on the glycemic scale, another important attribute in AGE prevention.

Buckwheat has been found to actually inhibit AGE formation on collagen thanks to its high rutin content. Rutin is a flavonoid that is also present in black tea and apple peels; however, buckwheat is a particularly rich source of this antioxidant. This remarkable finding means that we can safely consider buckwheat a powerful anti-aging, anti–skin wrinkling food, one worthy of regular consumption.

Another positive attribute of buckwheat is that it is gluten free, making it a safe choice for people with gluten allergy or celiac disease. It also contains more protein than rice, wheat, millet, or corn, and is high in the essential amino acids lysine and arginine, which are lacking in most grains.

Additional Buckwheat Benefits

- Compared to true grains, buckwheat is higher in vitamins and minerals.

- Buckwheat has up to 100% more calcium than other grains, is rich in vitamin E, and contains almost the entire range of B-complex vitamins. It also contains monounsaturated fatty acids, the same fats that give olive oil its healthy profile.

- It is a great source of soluble fiber, helping reduce cholesterol and lower the risk of colon cancer.

- It is high in Resistant Starch (RS), which is important in colon health and the reduction of blood sugar.

- It substantially reduces blood-glucose levels, partly due to rare carbohydrate compounds known as fagopyritols (especially D-chiroinositol), of which buckwheat is by far the *richest food source* yet discovered.

- It reduces high blood pressure and LDL (bad) cholesterol, and discourages obesity. Most recently, a buckwheat extract substantially reduced blood-glucose levels in diabetic rats, a promising finding that should lead to similar research in human diabetics.

GARDEN OF EATIN'

Nature's verdant farmlands and fruit-filled orchards provide us with AGE and age-preventing bounty. All the fruits and vegetables listed below are high in antioxidants, fiber, vitamins, and minerals. They are low in fat and/or contain healthy fats, and will not promote the formation of AGEs.

Because they have anti-inflammatory activity, they also help quench the AGE-generated inflammation in all organ systems.

Apples

Artichokes

Arugula

Asparagus

Avocados

Bamboo Shoots

Blueberries, blackberries, strawberries, raspberries (and all other
berries)

Bok Choy

Broccoli

Broccoli rabe

Brussels sprouts

Cabbage

Cauliflower

Celeriac

Celery

Cherries

Chicory

Chinese cabbage

Citrus fruits

Collard Greens

Cranberries

Cucumbers

Dandelion greens

Dark green leafy lettuces (baby
greens)

Eggplant

Endive

Escarole

Grapefruit

Green beans

Greens (turnip, collard, mustard,
dark lettuce)

Jerusalem artichokes

Kale

Lemons

Melons (all types)

Mushrooms

Onions (including garlic, chives,
leeks, scallions, green onions, shallots)

Pea pods

Pears

Peppers (green, red, orange, yellow;
also hot peppers)

Radishes

Rutabagas

Sea vegetables (kelp, nori, arami,
hijiki, wakame, dulse, kombu)

Spinach

Sprouts (all kinds)

Summer squash

Swiss chard

Tomatoes

Turnips

Water chestnuts

Watercress

Winter squash

Zucchini

Fruits and Fructose

Because fructose occurs naturally in fruit, many people think it is a more healthful choice than sugar. However, when it is in the fruit, it is bound to its fiber, nutrients, and vitamins. This means that for the most part, the small quantity of fructose in the fruit will be absorbed slowly because it is released slowly into the bloodstream.

When fructose is added to foods in the same way that cane sugar is, however, the opposite becomes true. Fructose is then rapidly absorbed into the bloodstream, creating a host of problems. In addition, fructose is particularly adept at combining with amino acids to form AGEs. High fructose intake has been shown to contribute to increased glycation throughout the body.

BLOCK OF AGES: HERBS AND SPICES

Along with fruits and vegetables (including beans and legumes), herbs and spices form the cornerstone of anti-AGEs foods and supplements thanks in part to their powerful anti-inflammatory activity. This is of tremendous importance because AGEs are veritable factories, generating hugely damaging inflammation to all organ systems. But herbs and spices also provide a double whammy to AGEs because they have exceptional abilities to lower blood sugar and increase insulin sensitivity. But perhaps most important, they are what make ordinary foods into special treats to delight the palate and help turn a healthy meal into an enticing one. It might seem hard to believe that as small an amount as ¼ teaspoon can pack such a punch to both the palate and the physical body. However, when it comes to herbs and spices, it's true. These roots, barks, and leaves are as potent as they are pungent. Ounce for ounce, they have more AGE-preventive powers than all other foods. Here is a list of our most popular herbs and spices, many of which can be used either fresh or dried.

Allspice

Anise

Basil

Bay leaf

Caraway seeds

Cardamom

Cayenne

Celery seed

Chervil

Chili flakes

Chives

Cilantro

Cinnamon (sticks, whole bark, ground)

Clove

Coriander

Cumin

Curry

Dill seed

Dill weed

Fennel

Fenugreek seed

Garam masala

Garlic

Ginger (root, ground)

Herbs de Provence

Juniper berries

Lemon balm

Lemon grass

Lemon peel

Lemon zest

Mace

Marjoram

Mint

Mustard powder

Mustard seed

Nutmeg

Oregano

Paprika (sweet and hot)

Parsley

Peppercorns (black, green, white, pink)

Poppyseed

Red pepper flakes

Rosemary

Saffron

Sage

Savory

Sea salt

Sesame seed

Star anise

Tarragon

Turmeric

Thyme

Vanilla bean

Don't Forget the Turmeric!

Two spices with outstanding anti-inflammatory and antioxidant activity are turmeric and cinnamon. They are covered in depth in Chapter Three, and their health and anti-AGEs benefits are legion, so use them liberally in your dishes.

LIQUID GOLD

Water is the most consumed beverage in the world, and most experts agree that eight glasses a day is a minimum requirement. Tea is the second-most-consumed beverage, and the good news is that it is packed with antioxidants and can be used, along with or instead of water, to fulfill your fluid requirements for the day. Substances in green tea have also been found to block starch absorption—important in blocking AGE formation.

Here is a list of healthful beverages.

Organic green tea

Organic white tea

Organic black tea

Water (pure spring water like Fiji or Poland Spring)

Acai pulp (Sambazon has unsweetened products; see Resources section)

Pomegranate juice (unsweetened)

Cocoa (made with pure cocoa powder and stevia or agave)

Red wine (in moderation)

Herbal teas

SWEET TREATS

See Chapter Two to learn about the hidden sugars in foods. Avoid artificial sweeteners of all kinds. Luckily, the choices below allow you to enjoy the sweetness you love without sacrificing your health.

Best Sweetener Choices

Stevia is a naturally sweet plant native to Paraguay that, in its unprocessed form, is 30 times sweeter than sugar. Stevia appears to be a good choice for a natural sweetener that will not promote AGE formation.

Agave is a honey-like syrup with a low glycemic index. Made from Mexico's Blue Agave cactus (the same plant from which tequila is made), agave sweetens naturally without spiking blood sugar.

Honey is all natural, and has been around for thousands of years. Honey comes in at 55 on the glycemic index. Although experts recommend keeping your food choices under 50 on the glycemic index, 55 is not bad for a sweetener.

HEALTHY FATS AND OILS

Organic extra-virgin olive oil (look for high-quality Italian or Spanish brands)

Flax oil

Grape seed oil

Macadamia nut oil

Avocados

Coconuts

Olives

Nuts and seeds

CONDIMENTS

Salsa (no added sweetener)

Fruit-sweetened ketchup such as Westbrae

Unsweetened "UnKetchup" from Westbrae

Mustard (sugar and preservative free)

Marinades (e.g., Vital Choice (www.vitalchoice.com). See Chapter Eleven for excellent marinade recipes.

All-natural spice rubs for meat

Westbrae is a company with some great condiments; its products are available at Whole Foods and Wild Oats. If you are vegetarian, you can safely choose their products, as Westbrae Natural does not use any animal products except for cream powder and butter in soups, and these are clearly listed in the ingredients. For more information, visit *www.westbrae.com.* Wild Oats and Whole Foods also offer their own brands of all-natural condiments.

GENERAL DOS AND DON'TS FOR ANTI-AGEs EATING

Do:

- Incorporate liquid into your dishes, gently steaming, poaching, or cooking in marinades.

- Cut proteins (fish, poultry, tofu) into small pieces for stir-fries so that cooking time is reduced.

- Cook protein foods such as meat in liquids—this will infuse them with the flavor of the sauce and keep AGE formation down.

- Marinate first if you grill or barbecue.

▨ Enjoy soups and stews, which are great ways to enjoy protein and veggies—just remember to gently simmer and not overcook to retain nutrients.

▨ Enjoy a wide variety of raw, organic vegetables and fruits—wash and dry them first. Even though there should be no pesticide residue, there is great concern about the E. coli breakouts associated with food handlers and packers of many fruits and vegetables.

▨ Remember that the highest AGE levels are found in animal products high in protein and saturated fat, such as meats. Fatty fish and grass-fed beef contain healthy fats that do not promote AGEs.

▨ Remember when sautéing foods such as onions and garlic to cook until just transparent rather than browned.

▨ Choose skinless poultry to keep fat levels down.

▨ Choose meat that has been grass fed as opposed to corn fed for a much healthier profile and much less saturated fat.

Don't:

▨ Choose processed meats such as hot dogs and bacon, which contain high AGE levels.

▨ Eat foods high in saturated or trans fats (regardless of how they are cooked) due to increased risk of diabetes.

▨ Eat charred or blackened foods.

▨ Fry or deep-fry foods—we need to stay away from very high heat

▨ Cook at extreme heats or for long periods of time.

▨ Dredge meat in flour before sautéing because flour is high glycemic and it increases AGE formation. This is a classic example of the sugar–amino acid–heat connection in AGEs.

For delicious recipes made with recommended ingredients and cooking methods, see Chapter Eleven.

The Simple Life

The best advice is to avoid foods that are highly processed and prepackaged, as they usually have added flavors, preservatives, and colors. Keep your food choices pure and simple. If you're buying packaged, canned, or bottled foods, read the labels and avoid those with chemical ingredients. Packaged, canned, and bottled foods that have few ingredients (e.g., tomato paste, which is made from just tomatoes and salt, or canned beans containing beans, water, and salt) are fine. If you have to be a rocket scientist to figure out what is in that can, it is not going to be a good choice. To avoid chemical ingredients and ensure that your foods have the highest levels of nutrients, purchase fresh food. Frozen food is acceptable as long as its ingredients are simple, such as frozen vegetables, fruits, or fish. Beware of frozen meals regardless of whether they have "Healthy" in their name—these are often the direct opposite of healthy.

In general, if you are buying brands that say "organic" and "all natural," the foods must be refrigerated and used in a timely manner because they don't contain the preservatives, stabilizers, and so forth found in processed foods. Read all labels, and avoid foods and condiments that contain sugar, high-fructose corn syrup, MSG, salt, preservatives, food coloring, and other undesirable ingredients as outlined in Chapter Two.

In the next chapter, you will learn about the role of nutritional supplements in preventing AGEs and helping mitigate their damaging effects. New research has provided exciting categories of supplements, vastly improving on existing technology to help us lower blood sugar, slow or impede AGE formation, and even block the absorption of sugars and starches, allowing us the occasional opportunity to have our cake and eat it too.

PART THREE

Nutritional Supplements to Reverse AGEs

5

The Abcs of Anti-AGEs Supplements

am starting this chapter with two of the very best nutrients for preventing and helping to reverse the effects of AGEs. They were first introduced in *The Perricone Promise* as part of a triple crown of antiglycating agents consisting of alpha lipoic acid, benfotiamine, and carnosine. Alpha lipoic acid, for example, gets rid of the host of free radicals that are generated by AGEs. And it is also a powerful antiglycating nutrient in its own right. Benfotiamine, long revered as an antidiabetic drug in Europe, is finally being recognized in the U.S. for its outstanding ability to prevent AGE-related diseases and degenerative conditions in the nondiabetic population. When it comes to carnosine, a fascinating laboratory breakthrough has accelerated its AGE-fighting prowess, earning it its very own chapter (see Chapter Six).

I am happy to report that important new research not only continues to validate the efficacy of these supplements, but also expands upon their usefulness. Yet very few people are aware of their existence, let alone their power as anti-aging nutrients. While they are indispensable cornerstones of the anti-AGEs program, I also introduce other powerful nutri-

ents in this chapter that work in a variety of ways to counteract the debilitating effects of AGE formation. One of them, known as a starch blocker,
can actually head off carbohydrates at the pass—that is, neutralize or block
carbohydrate digestion, thus blocking the carbs' ability to raise blood
sugar. This remarkable substance can even be used in products such as
pasta, enabling us to occasionally enjoy foods that are normally implicated in raising blood-sugar and insulin levels.

The SX fraction of maitake mushroom is another powerful AGEs
blocker. Countless studies have shown this remarkable mushroom to be
truly magic, as it is extremely effective in maintaining healthy blood-
sugar levels and preventing insulin resistance—two critical strategies to
prevent AGEs. Another nutrient, one that has been attracting a great deal
of scientific scrutiny, is chromium. The Western diet is notoriously deficient in this critical trace mineral, which plays a tremendously important
role in preventing sugar's damaging effects in the body. Ironically, diets
high in sugar deplete chromium, compounding the problem.

ALPHA LIPOIC ACID

Alpha lipoic acid (ALA) is a tremendously important, broad-spectrum
antioxidant that has a powerful ability to counteract the effects of AGEs.
In fact, ALA has long been known to be one of the few proven antiglycating agents, making it a very significant anti-aging supplement. We know
that one of the detrimental effects of AGEs is their ability to continuously
generate inflammation. Because ALA is both fat and water soluble, it is
able to quench a wide range of inflammation-producing free radicals. It
also has the unique ability to recycle itself, as well as other important antioxidants including vitamins C and E, glutathione, and coenzyme Q-10.
This is a significant and critical function because when AGEs are formed,
the inflammation-generated oxidative stress they cause rapidly depletes
these important nutrients. This will then accelerate the breakdown of all
organ systems. For these reasons, ALA is called the *universal antioxidant*.
It is 400 times more effective than vitamin C and E combined. Remember
this very noteworthy fact: ALA literally mops up many of the free radicals
generated by AGEs, and prevents them from destroying the body on a cellular level.

ALA: The Antioxidant Booster

ALA is the only antioxidant that can boost the level of glutathione, a cellular tripeptide antioxidant of tremendous importance. For an in-depth look at glutathione see Chapter Seven. Glutathione is essential for optimal functioning of the immune system; it is also the body's primary water-soluble antioxidant and a major detoxification agent. Because white blood cells are extremely sensitive to even small changes in glutathione levels, increases in glutathione have profound effects on our immune response. High glutathione levels are present in healthy older people, while people with chronic illnesses such as AIDS, cancer, and autoimmune diseases generally have very low levels. Like so many important substances, glutathione levels decline as we age. Therefore, maintaining high glutathione levels is a must if we are going to fight off the ravages of AGEs that accumulate over the years. Supplementation with ALA enables us to do this.

In addition, much of the damage associated with Alzheimer's disease is caused by a type of AGEs known as dicarbonyls. Fortunately, the human brain has an enzyme system that eliminates these AGEs. In order to function properly, however, this system requires glutathione. Unfortunately, AGE-generated free radical–induced inflammation interferes with the enzyme system's ability to eliminate the AGEs. Supplementation with ALA—which regenerates and elevates the depleted glutathione—indirectly strengthens the brain's antiglycation/anti-AGE defense system.

ALA Fights Diabetes

In addition to its ability to increase glutathione, quench AGE-generated, free radical–induced inflammation, recycle antioxidants, and chelate metals such as copper, ALA has also been shown to be beneficial in the prevention and treatment of diabetes.

ALA is necessary to convert dietary carbohydrates to energy in cells' mitochondria. It also helps prevent glycation by stimulating glucose uptake. In other words, ALA enhances the transfer of sugar out of the bloodstream and into the cells, where it can be used for energy. This reduces the amount of free glucose circulating in the blood and available for creating damaging AGE reactions. This is another strong link in the chain that ALA weaves in preventing AGEs and AGE-related damage.

U.S. Recommended Daily Intake (RDI): None established

Perricone Recommendation: 200 mg per day, in two doses of 100 mg (one at breakfast and one at dinner).

BENFOTIAMINE

This strange-sounding, little-known supplement deserves a place of honor in everyone's medicine cabinet. Benfotiamine is a synthetic, fat-soluble, highly absorbable form of vitamin B_1 (thiamine). A powerful anti-AGE agent, benfotiamine was first developed in Japan in the late 1950s to treat painful nerve conditions, including sciatica and neuropathy in alcoholics. Neuropathy is a disorder of the peripheral nerves—the motor, sensory, and autonomic nerves that connect the spinal cord to muscles, skin, and internal organs. Approximately 30% of neuropathies are "idiopathic," or of an unknown cause. In another 30% of cases, the cause is diabetes. Interestingly, researchers have found a direct link between neuropathy and AGEs, and have been searching for effective antiglycation agents to prevent and treat this condition. Benfotiamine assists on two fronts: It effectively treats neuropathy and blocks AGE formation.

As you have learned in this book, elevated blood sugar exacerbates the formation of AGEs. Benfotiamine works by blocking three of the major biochemical pathways through which hyperglycemia (high blood sugar) does its pro-inflammatory damage, including the formation of AGEs. In other words, benfotiamine prevents sugar and high-glycemic carbohydrates from creating glycation.

Benfotiamine not only blocks inflammation pathways, it also enhances the activity of an enzyme called transketolase, which (like ALA) prevents activation of the pro-inflammatory transcription factor NF-κB. AGEs act as inflammation factories, wreaking great havoc. By stimulating transketolase, benfotiamine stops the production of this inflammation. And there is even more good news. Benfotiamine also converts harmful blood-sugar metabolites (products that result from the breakdown of glucose in the body) into harmless chemicals, thereby preventing them from forming AGEs. Benfotiamine also helps the digestion process, enabling the body to properly use carbohydrates.

Although the traditional water-soluble form of vitamin B₁ also works to moderate the damage caused by high blood-sugar levels, fat-soluble benfotiamine does it better, and in smaller doses. Benfotiamine also shows promise in treating a number of neurological and vascular conditions. And it appears to have beneficial anti-aging qualities, protecting human cells from harmful metabolic end products.

Benfotiamine can also improve mental attitude. It helps with all types of physical and mental stress, so the need for this vitamin increases when one is anxious and during illness, trauma, and postsurgical periods.

Women who are pregnant, nursing, or taking birth control pills have increased needs for vitamin B₁. Smokers, people who drink alcohol, and those who consume a great deal of sugar or caffeine, all implicated in AGE formation, are also advised to increase their intake of vitamin B₁—ideally in the form of fat-soluble benfotiamine as opposed to water-soluble thiamine because it is much easier to achieve therapeutic doses.

Benfotiamine occurs naturally in foods of the allium family, such as garlic, onions, shallots, scallions, and leeks—another significant health benefit and reason to enjoy these vegetables, which also add great flavor to every dish. Benfotiamine is also a very safe supplement. Standard thiamine (Vitamin B₁) shows no adverse effects even at high doses (several hundred milligrams a day), and safety tests indicate that benfotiamine is even safer.

U.S. Recommended Daily Intake (RDI): None established

Perricone Recommendation: 300 mg per day (150 mg at breakfast and 150 mg at dinner) for 30 days and then one capsule per day thereafter or as directed by your physician.

CARBOHYDRATE (STARCH) BLOCKER

Carbohydrate (starch) blockers comprise an exciting new category. They are not a new idea, but what is new is that they now actually work. The dream of the 1970s, to effectively block the absorption of carbohydrates, is now a reality.

Starch blockers represent a very important breakthrough in finding ways to block the damage caused by AGE formation. Although we know that sugar and refined carbohydrates are the major causes of AGEs, we still succumb to that occasional bagel, doughnut, pasta dish, soda, or slice of pizza. With the new starch blockers, we have what appears to be a safe and effective version of a concept that has been around for decades. Here is how they work.

During the digestive process, your body converts carbohydrates—found in starchy foods such as potatoes, bread, and pasta—into sugar by breaking down the carbohydrate molecule with alpha amylase, an enzyme that is produced in the pancreas. These sugar calories are then either burned off through exercise or stored in fat cells for future use. Unfortunately, inactivity means that these stored fat cells increase in size. The result is weight gain.

Phase 2 Starch Neutralizer®, an exclusive, all-natural nutritional ingredient extracted from white kidney beans, "neutralizes" some of the digestive enzyme alpha amylase before it can convert starch into sugar and then fat. Essentially, it allows some of the starchy carbohydrates to pass through the system with less caloric intake.

This is the first nutritional ingredient that has been clinically and scientifically proven to neutralize the starch found in many of our favorite foods such as potatoes, breads, pasta, rice, corn, and crackers. Taking Phase 2 as a supplement allows us to enjoy these foods (in moderation) while cutting back on starch and glucose absorption.

Putting It to the Test

Along with Dr. Harry Preuss at Georgetown University Medical Center, I reviewed the findings and co-wrote the research with the original investigators for the study "A Dietary Supplement Containing Standardized Phaseolus vulgaris Extract Influences Body Composition of Overweight Men and Women," which was published in the January 2007 issue of the *International Journal of Medical Sciences*.

The study was conducted at the Cosmetic Research Center, dell'Universita Cattolica di Roma in Rome, Italy by L. Celleno, M. V. Tolaini, and A. D'Amore. The study involved 60 healthy human volunteers, both males and females, ranging in age from 20 to 45 years old. The participants were selected based on being anywhere from 5 to 15 kg (11 to 33 pounds) over-weight for at least six months.

Participants were divided into two groups of 30, with one group receiving a placebo and the other receiving the placebo plus 500 mg of Phase 2 in a product called Blockal. Neither the participants nor the study administrators knew who received the placebo and who received the Phase 2.

The exciting results of this investigation showed that, when taken daily by overweight humans with the carbohydrate-rich portion of a 2000- to 2200-calorie diet, a dietary formula containing Phaseolus vulgaris extract (Phase 2®) as the major ingredient produced significant decreases in body fat while essentially maintaining lean body mass.

Participants in the double-blind study lost an average of 6.45 pounds in 30 days when they consumed Phase 2. Participants on the placebo lost less than one pound on average. In addition, participants on Phase 2 lost 10.45% of fat body mass, 1.39% in hip circumference, 1.44% in thigh circumference, and 3.44% in waist circumference. These losses were experienced without any loss of lean body mass. The observed differences were statistically significant for all test parameters.

I concluded from the results of the study that these "starch blockers" may indeed promote weight loss by interfering with the breakdown of complex carbohydrates, thereby reducing, or at least slowing, the digestive availability of carbohydrate-derived calories. This could become a major tool in our goal to reduce glycemic response from carbohydrates.

More Pasta, Fewer Carbs

Many commercially prepared food manufacturers are beginning to offer a lower–glycemic index version of their products, including a pasta known as Carbolina™. Carbolina was created by Italian-born, Chicago-based chef Charles Galletta in response to orders from his physician to give up regular pasta because his blood-sugar levels were dangerously high. He harnessed the passion for cooking he had developed in more than 40 years in the restaurant business to experiment with recipes that would reduce the absorption of starch in his favorite foods. He selected the white bean extract, which has been clinically shown to delay the digestion and absorption of carbohydrates, while also reducing the glycemic index and (GI) caloric impact of starchy foods. Chef Galletta developed a number of pasta recipes until he was satisfied with the taste and texture. He then compared his new pasta to regular pasta to determine its impact on his blood-sugar levels.

"I discovered that the new recipes tasted great, and my glucose would return to normal much faster," says Chef Galletta. "With the other pastas my blood glucose would go up and stay there until I took my medication."

Carbolina allows us to enjoy an occasional side dish of pasta by providing us with an alternative to traditional pasta, one that will not cause dangerous swings in blood sugar and insulin.

Make sure you eat a fiber-rich salad with chickpeas or lentils to accompany the pasta so that you are increasing your "carb insurance," as well as getting that all-important fiber—remember, beans and lentils lower blood sugar and continue to do so into the next meal as well—regardless of whether that meal contains beans or lentils.

More of a Good Thing

In addition to the white bean extract described on page 101, a number of natural products can influence glucose absorption by other mechanisms. For instance, when isolated, L-arabinose, a carbohydrate found naturally in foods such as beets and corn, blocks the activity of the gastrointestinal enzyme *sucrase*, whose job is to break sucrose down into glucose and fructose so that they can be utilized by the body. If sucrose *cannot* be broken down into glucose and fructose, then it is not readily absorbed—and if it can't be absorbed it can't turn into fat, nor can it cause glycation or AGE formation—very exciting news. In other words, if the enzyme *sucrase* is blocked from converting *sucrose* into glucose and fructose, sucrose can't be absorbed and is essentially rendered harmless. Because of this, research has found that L-arabinose can help prevent obesity and type 2 diabetes (which are exacerbated by a diet high in sugars and starches), by blocking the absorption of sugars and starches. Specifically, an animal experiment confirmed that a 19-week administration of L-arabinose prevents weight gain and reduces the rise of both the fasting blood-sugar level and the insulin-resistance index.

Hibiscus flower extract (*Hibiscus sabdariffa*), green tea leaf extract (*Camellia sinensis*), and apple extract (*Malus silvestris*) have all also been reported to impede the gastrointestinal absorption of starch. A supplement known as Carb-Ease™ has been studied by Dr. Preuss at Georgetown with excellent results. Carb-Ease helps prevent the breakdown of carbohydrates by inhibiting the digestive enzymes used to break them down. Carb-Ease contains dry bean extract, hibiscus extract, green tea extract, apple extract, L-arabinose, and additional ingredients that help lessen the absorption of sugars and starches before they are stored and converted to fat. To find out where to purchase Carb-Ease, Phase 2, and Carbolina products check the Resources section at the back of the book.

GARLIC AND AGED GARLIC EXTRACT

Garlic, an antioxidant plant, is the edible bulb of a plant in the lily family. Garlic dates back at least 6,000 years, and has been a popular and delicious staple worldwide. Now we can also add it to the list of natural substances that can prevent AGE formation due to its positive impact on blood sugar.

Garlic can be used raw or cooked, and offers many health benefits, including the following, which are listed on the National Institutes of Health's website. Garlic may

- slow the development of atherosclerosis. As you learned in the section on omega-3s, the development of atherosclerosis—the leading cause of heart disease—is the result of AGE formation

- lower blood-cholesterol levels

- reduce risk factors for cardiovascular diseases and cancer

- stimulate immune function

- enhance the body's ability to detoxify foreign substances

- restore physical strength

- increase resistance to a wide variety of stresses

■ provide anti-aging effects

■ act as an antioxidant

■ protect the liver

In addition to using garlic to treat hypercholesterolemia (chronically high levels of cholesterol in the blood), and hypertension (high blood pressure), garlic can also help lower blood sugar. This is very important in protecting against AGEs. An interesting study using aged garlic extract found that garlic has a statistically significant effect in inhibiting or decreasing the reaction of glycation. The study proved that garlic lowers the blood-glucose level by increasing the body's circulating insulin, and by increasing glycogen storage in the liver, where it can supply the body with energy.

Perricone Recommendation: Take two 300-mg aged garlic extract capsules with a meal twice per day.

MAITAKE SX FRACTION

Maitake SX Fraction is an excellent supplement that helps prevent the formation of AGEs by controlling blood-sugar and insulin levels. One of the leading experts in this field is my friend and colleague Harry G. Preuss, M.D. Dr. Preuss is the highly respected author of the book *Maitake Magic*, as well as coauthor of a number of scientific studies on maitake.

Maitake contains the highly beneficial polysaccharides known as beta-glucans mentioned on page 80, which have been shown in both laboratory and clinical studies to have a wide range of immune-stimulating and protective effects within the body. Maitake also lowers cholesterol, reduces high blood pressure, and aids weight loss. Remember the importance of excess weight as a contributing factor to AGE formation.

Three of the important recurring themes in my choice of supplements for AGE prevention are the maintenance of healthy blood-sugar and insulin levels and increasing insulin sensitivity. In this way the cells can properly use the sugar and insulin. This is one of the single most important steps we can take in stopping the glycation of proteins that occurs with AGEs. Much research has been done with Grifon Maitake

SX-Fraction®, which is a proprietary and innovative form of this mushroom. It is the only product standardized to contain the bioactive ingredient that can counter various chronic disorders caused by the malfunction of insulin and sugar metabolism—including metabolic syndrome, diabetes, and AGE formation. We need to properly metabolize sugar and fats for AGE prevention, and maitake SX fraction does this and more. Maitake SX Fraction:

- Supports healthy insulin function.

- Promotes healthy sugar metabolism.

- Supports healthy lipid (fat) metabolism.

- Supports healthy body-weight management.

- Maintains healthy blood-sugar levels.

- Maintains healthy cardiovascular function.

Perricone Recommendation: 300 mg per day, in three doses of 100 mg between meals or as directed by your physician.

NIACIN-BOUND CHROMIUM

Niacin-bound chromium (NBC) is a little-known, little-understood, and underutilized supplement that offers significant health, anti-AGEs, anti-obesity, antidiabetes, and anti-aging benefits. But first a little history to better understand this unique substance. Like maitake mushroom, chromium also helps prevent metabolic syndrome (the hormonal problem created by a diet high in sugars and starches), which interferes with the body's ability to efficiently burn food. As we know, once ingested, sugars and starches are turned into glucose, the form in which all carbohydrates are used as the body's principal energy source. Ideally, the glucose is transported in the blood and metabolized in the tissues. However, the chronically high levels of sugars and starches in the Western diet have led to the current obesity and diabetes epidemic. When our bodies cannot effectively use glucose, the result is glycation and AGE formation, causing

a host of diseases as well as accelerated aging. Because our culture is so in-
undated with high-glycemic foods, it is unrealistic to believe that people
will give them up completely. But the good news is that research shows
that taking niacin-bound chromium can help offset some of the negative
effects caused by eating simple sugars and refined starches. Ironically,
sugar and starches also deplete the body's natural store of chromium, so it
is all the more critical to take chromium as a supplement.

In the 1950s, Dr. Walter Mertz, a researcher at the U.S. Department of
Agriculture, found that animals fed chromium-deficient *torula* yeast developed diabetic-like symptoms. But when they were fed chromium-rich
brewer's yeast, the symptoms disappeared. Dr. Mertz's discovery led to the
identification of something known as Glucose Tolerance Factor (GTF), a
biologically active form of NBC that facilitates normal insulin function.

There are different forms of chromium, but it was Dr. Mertz who recognized the importance of the niacin-bound form. Niacin is part of the B-
vitamin complex, also known as vitamin B_3. It is crucial for the conversion
of food into energy, and it helps maintain normal functioning of the skin,
nerves, and digestive system. To prove the importance of niacin, Dr.
Mertz compared NBC with chromium bound to picolinic acid, an isomer
(molecules containing the same atoms but differently arranged) of niacin
that is nearly identical in chemical structure. Dr. Mertz showed that pure
NBC significantly increased insulin activity similar to the way that GTF
found in nature does, whereas chromium picolinate had no effect on insulin activity. I make this differentiation because there are many different types of chromium on the market, and it is important to know which
varieties have efficacy and are backed by scientific studies.

Extensive clinical and subclinical research has shown that the niacin-
bound form of chromium known as ChromeMate® is the superior form of
chromium. ChromeMate is a unique form of *oxygen-coordinated* NBC—
generically known as chromium nicotinate or chromium polynicotinate—
that dramatically increases the safety and efficacy of chromium. Research
has clearly demonstrated that this form of NBC provides significant
health benefits to those with diabetes or metabolic syndrome, including
the prevention of glycation leading to AGEs, and is, indeed, the optimal
form of chromium available as a dietary supplement. Studies have shown
the following benefits:

- Promotion of proper insulin function and normal blood-sugar levels;

- Promotion of healthy blood-cholesterol levels, normal blood pressure, and cardiovascular health; and

- Promotion of healthy body weight and lean body mass (building of muscle).

Recently we saw another very important benefit. ChromeMate was shown in animal studies to increase the average life span by 20% compared to animals taking a placebo. This is a very exciting discovery. Resveratrol and calorie restriction (CR) have so far been the only ways scientists have been able to measurably increase life span, as you will learn in Chapter Seven.

Furthermore, ChromeMate has consistently been shown to be safer and more effective than chromium picolinate.

- Researchers at the University of California, Davis, showed that in animal models used to evaluate bioavailability in humans ChromeMate was on average absorbed and retained more than 300% better than chromium picolinate and 600% better than chromium chloride. Other studies have shown that ChromeMate's unique complex is 18 times more bioactive than other forms of NBC.

- Researchers from Dartmouth College and George Washington University Medical Center found that ChromeMate did not cause chromosomal damage to hamster ovary cells, while chromium picolinate and picolinic acid did. This is important—read labels carefully and make sure the product you are purchasing contains the word ChromeMate, not other forms of chromium that do not have ChromeMate's safety profile.

- Researchers at the University of Texas, Austin, showed that a combination of ChromeMate plus exercise in obese women resulted in significant loss of body weight and improved insulin function, while chromium picolinate did not. In fact, the study found that chromium picolinate without exercise resulted in significant *weight gain*, which is, as we know, directly linked to obesity, accelerated aging, metabolic syndrome, and accelerated AGE formation. You will notice that many of the nutrients recommended as AGE preventive are also important in contributing to healthy weight maintenance and weight loss.

■ Researchers at Georgetown University Medical Center showed that both ChromeMate and chromium picolinate significantly inhibit sugar-induced high blood pressure, improve long-term blood-sugar status, and reduce liver lipid peroxidation in rats. However, ChromeMate also significantly reduced kidney lipid peroxidation, while chromium picolinate did not. That is, ChromeMate protects fats in both the liver and the kidney from free radical degradation, while chromium picolinate did only the former.

In addition to its extensive proven efficacy, ChromeMate has been affirmed GRAS (Generally Recognized as Safe, a standard of safety for food and beverage ingredients) by the Burdock Group, the nation's leading toxicology specialists in evaluating the safety of food and beverage ingredients. This GRAS affirmation is based on the results of extensive safety studies, including acute oral, acute dermal, primary dermal, and eye irritation; genotoxicity; 90-day subchronic toxicity; and human studies, as well as its long history of use as a safe and effective dietary supplement. A supplement as important as NBC should be in everyone's cupboard.

Perricone Recommendation: 100 mcg (micrograms) once a day

The Grape Seed Extract Boost

As mentioned, there have been many important studies conducted on the anti-aging effects of NBC, specifically on the ChromeMate brand. In one study particularly relevant to this book, Dr. Harry Preuss and colleagues found that the combination of NBC and grape seed extract (GSE) was highly effective in reducing damage from free radicals, disturbances in the insulin-glucose system, and other age-related risk factors. Several important animal studies have shown that ChromeMate, alone or when combined with grape seed extract, reduces biomarkers of oxidative stress. This combination reduces the inflammation caused by AGE-generated free radicals, lowers blood pressure in normal and hypertensive rats, and enhances insulin action in rats with normal blood pressure. These studies suggest that both NBC and GSE lower oxidative stress and systolic blood pressure in rats with normal blood pressure. In human clinical studies, NBC supplementation reduced body fat and spared lean muscle mass in overweight African-American women, and was shown to decrease LDL cholesterol levels in double-blind, placebo-controlled trials of subjects with elevated cholesterol. The authors of these studies concluded that ChromeMate and grape seed extract can favorably alter risk factors associated with metabolic syndrome and aging—important news for the prevention of AGE formation.

Perricone Recommendation: NBC, 100 mcg (micrograms) once per day. GSE, 125 mg (milligrams), one to three capsules daily

OMEGA-3 ESSENTIAL FATTY ACIDS

The myriad of benefits of the omega-3 essential fatty acids never ceases to amaze me, and each day new studies appear supporting the critical need to include these healthy fats in our diets. I include the omega-3s as a supplement in this chapter but want to make it clear that this information also applies to omega-3–rich foods, such as salmon, trout, herring, sardines, anchovies, and other cold-water fish, and to a lesser extent to nuts and seeds. Omega-3s are also extremely important in treating and reversing obesity, which is part of the metabolic syndrome and a precursor to both heart disease and diabetes.

Omega-3 Puts the Brake on Diabetes

Research published in recent years supports the idea that inflammation, obesity, and diabetes are interconnected, and highlights the fact that a diet rich in omega-3s can discourage all three.

A new animal study from the Medical University of Vienna, Austria underscores these connections and supports the hypothesis that marine omega-3s can help prevent or ameliorate type 2 diabetes. This is an extremely important finding, as it means that omega-3s can also help prevent or ameliorate glycation and AGE formation.

As I stress, the fat that accumulates around people's waists and abdomens results in dangerous "central obesity." This type of fat attracts immune system cells (macrophages) that generate a steady stream of the kinds of pro-inflammatory messenger chemicals (e.g., cytokines and prostaglandins) normally generated only in response to injury, cancer, or infection.

Increases in the proportion of adipose tissue (fat) in the body also reduce the insulin sensitivity of cells, the first step in a long chain of events that results in obesity, the breakdown of muscle tissue, diabetes, and AGEs.

As the authors of the Austrian study found, this abdominal body fat is responsible for many of the health problems related to obesity, including diabetes. Fortunately, they also found that polyunsaturated fatty acids, especially omega-3 essential fatty acids, had a favorable effect on the immune system and helped offset the decreased insulin sensitivity caused by the body fat. They tested this hypothesis by feeding overweight diabetic mice either a low-fat diet or one of three diets:

1. A high-fat diet dominated by saturated and monounsaturated fatty acids.

2. A high-fat omega-6 diet (dominated by pro-inflammatory omega-6 fatty acids such as those found in most vegetable oils—corn, soy, safflower, etc.)

3. A high-fat omega-3 diet (dominated by anti-inflammatory omega-3 fatty acids from fish).

The Austrians reported that the diabetic mice on high-fat diet number 1 (saturated and monounsaturated fatty acids) suffered two adverse effects, compared with the diabetic mice on the low-fat diet:

1. Increased cellular inflammation, which breaks down the cell (we need intact cells to remain disease free)

2. Their body fat itself began to generate AGE-mediated inflammatory compounds. This is important because it demonstrates a truly vicious cycle. Our stored fat cells act as a veritable factory for creating inflammatory chemicals, which increase inflammation. This increased inflammation further inhibits insulin and glucose utilization. The result? Increased AGE formation and the accumulation of additional excess fat.

Unsurprisingly, the mice on high-fat diet number 2, rich in proinflammatory omega-6 fatty acids, suffered similar adverse, proinflammatory effects in their adipose (fat) tissues.

However, the diabetic mice on the high-fat omega-3 diet avoided all of the negative, pro-inflammatory effects suffered by the other two high-fat groups, despite the fact that their body weight did not drop.

Another benefit for the mice fed the omega-3 diet related to their body mass index (BMI). The hormone known as adiponectin, which affects BMI, remained high. However, it was significantly reduced in the mice on high-fat diets 1 and 2. Adiponectin is produced and secreted exclusively by fat cells. It regulates the metabolism of lipids and glucose, and influences the body's response to insulin. High levels enable our cells to properly use fats, glucose, and insulin, thereby preventing AGE formation.

When we look at a list of some of the benefits accrued from a diet rich in omega-3s, we can see how they counteract the effects of an AGE-promoting diet, which destabilizes blood sugar and insulin, increases body fat, decreases muscle mass, increases mental confusion and depression, alters serotonin, increases fatigue, and so forth.

Where Have All the Omega-3s Gone?

The tremendous decline in the intake of omega-3s has multiple causes, including modern farming and animal husbandry methods. Commercial beef and dairy products no longer contain omega-3 fatty acids, as they once did. When cows are in the pasture eating grass (their natural diet) their milk and meat contain high levels of this important nutrient. Instead, modern agriculture raises them on corn, a significant source of omega-6 fatty acids, upsetting the natural balance. We know that omega-3 may help prevent many cancers, including breast cancer. Conversely, a new study recently published in the *British Journal of Cancer* finds that postmenopausal women who eat even a small amount of meat daily—even as little as two ounces of beef, pork, or lamb—face a 56% increased risk of breast cancer compared to those who abstain. The study examined approximately 35,000 women between the ages of 35 and 69 for eight years. Meanwhile, those who eat more than 3.6 ounces of processed meat a day, such as bacon, sausages, or meat pies, had an even greater—64%—risk of developing the disease.

Grass-fed beef is up to three times leaner than grain-fed beef, and can have up to 15 fewer calories per ounce than beef from a grain-fed cow. As mentioned, grass-fed meat and dairy also provide more-balanced omega-3s and omega-6s, which help guard against a variety of ailments.

Like wild salmon, grass-fed beef is an excellent source of high-quality omega-3 essential fatty acid, as well as conjugated linoleic acid (CLA). CLA has many benefits, including the protection of lean muscle mass and the reduction of body fat, especially in the abdominal area. However, with the cows' dietary change from grass to grain, levels of CLA dramatically decreased in meat and dairy products. It is no wonder we have such an epidemic of AGE-generated diseases; increased fat (especially in the abdominal area), diabetes, and heart disease; and accelerated aging.

When CLA is present in the food chain, it is found in the fatty portion of milk. Drinking skim milk prevents us from receiving the benefits of CLA. However, since CLA levels are now so low in animal products, skim versus full-fat milk is a moot point. Therefore, unless you are eating meat and dairy from grass-fed animals only, avoid full-fat dairy products and choose only the leanest cuts of meats—or better yet, avoid grain-fed beef and opt for organic, free-range poultry and wild fish. The lack of omega-3 and CLA have turned what were once healthy food choices into something quite different—potentially carcinogenic as well as promoting excess weight gain and disease-causing AGEs.

Omega-3 Blocks Fat

The link between body fat and AGEs is simple and direct. It is disturbances in glucose metabolism that result in fat storage, AGE formation,
cross-linking of proteins, inflammation, and free radical–generated oxidative stress. Even worse, once the fat has been formed, it can accelerate
the formation of even more fat cells, and can turn fat cells into a factory
for producing deadly inflammatory chemicals and accelerating AGE production. Thus, it is of the utmost importance to normalize our glucose
metabolism.

Although the problems of obesity and metabolic syndrome continue to
grow exponentially thanks to Western diets and lifestyles, we are fortunate to have many natural foods and supplements that have been proven
to help us prevent, stop, and reverse these negative effects.

Hye-Kyeong Kim and his colleagues at the University of Georgia report
that docosahexaenoic acid (DHA)—one of the two main omega-3s in fish
fat—interferes with the development of fat cells.

The purpose of Kim et al.'s study was to learn how increased intake of
omega-3 can result in reductions in abdominal fat, the risk of obesity,
and metabolic syndrome.

Previous animal studies had shown that omega-3s can reduce body fat,
block the development of fat cells, and actually aid weight management,
but the mechanism behind these effects was unclear.

The Georgia-based team examined the effects of DHA on cell growth,
cell differentiation, cell death (apoptosis), and fat breakdown in human
fat cells. When they added DHA to pre-adipocyte cells, which are cells
that can develop into fat cells (adipocytes), they recorded a reduction in
the number of fat cells that actually developed, even at the lowest levels of
added DHA. The researchers attributed this to DHA's ability to induce
cell death among the pre-adipocytes that could have become fat cells.
DHA was actually killing the cells before they could become full-fledged
fat cells.

The researchers also reported that DHA significantly decreased the accumulation of fat in the pre-adipocytes, and did it in a dose-dependent
manner that proved that the omega-3 was really responsible for the effect.

Omega-3 benefits include:

- stabilized blood-sugar levels

- lowered insulin levels

- reduced body fat

- maintenance of muscle mass

- elevated mood

- improved attention span

- promotion of healthy serotonin levels

- loss of the roller-coaster effects of carbohydrates

- decreased appetite

- increased skin radiance

- a healthier immune system

- increased energy levels

- decreased symptoms and severity of rheumatoid arthritis

- reduced symptoms and severity of chronic skin conditions such as eczema

- reduced blood levels of triglycerides (fat)

- increased blood levels of HDL ("good") cholesterol

- reduced blood pressure, inflammation, and stickiness of blood, thereby decreasing risk of heart disease

- improved performance of the endothelial tissues that line the arteries—important in preventing AGE-generated atherosclerosis, the leading cause of heart disease and stroke.

AGEs: At the Heart of Heart Disease

As you learned in Chapter Two, the many conditions that are defined as metabolic syndrome are risk factors for atherosclerosis and type 2 diabetes. While there isn't agreement on the precise parameters that push each of the factors that comprise metabolic syndrome into the danger zone, there is no disagreement that the syndrome is very real and is largely responsible for the epidemic of cardiovascular disease (CVD) and diabetes that's exploding throughout the developed and developing worlds. Fortunately, there is a growing body of evidence that indicates that fatty fish and omega-3 supplements may also help prevent or ameliorate metabolic syndrome, when combined with exercise and Mediterranean-style diets rich in beans, extra-virgin olive oil, and colorful vegetables.

It is no surprise to anyone that CVD is the leading cause of mortality worldwide. Because of this, getting a handle on preventing metabolic syndrome becomes increasingly important. CVD starts with atherosclerosis, what we used to refer to as hardening of the arteries, from the Greek words *athero* ("gruel" or "paste") and *sclerosis* ("hardness"). This definition is partially accurate but also a gross oversimplification.

Atherosclerosis, which is more aptly defined as the clogging, narrowing, and hardening of the body's large arteries and medium-sized blood vessels, can lead to stroke, heart attack, eye problems, and kidney problems, and is at the very heart of heart disease. We know that diabetics have more AGEs than nondiabetics, and that CVD is the leading cause of death for diabetics. However, the playing field appears to be leveled when it comes to the development of atherosclerosis, leading to CVD and the other problems listed above. In fact, there is now a large amount of evidence linking AGEs with the development and progression of atherosclerosis, regardless of diabetic status.

With CVD being the leading cause of death, finding strategies to prevent AGE formation should be one of the scientific community's top priorities. However, there have not been any significant, safe, and effective pharmacological therapies. This is why many scientists, physicians, and researchers, myself included, stress the importance of prevention, by avoiding sugars, high-glycemic starches, and processed, packaged foods as much as possible. In addition, fatty fish and fish oil should be important parts of our daily diet.

We know that people who eat a lot of fish—like the Japanese and Greenland's Inuit Eskimos—enjoy lower rates of many diseases, including heart disease and diabetes. There is ample evidence that diets high in fish or supplemental omega-3s can improve key cardiovascular functions and reduce major factors for heart disease, including metabolic syndrome. The American Dietetic Association recommends two to three servings of fish per week—advice echoed by the American Heart Association. I recommend even more for optimum health, especially with the recognition of the role that AGEs play in CVD. Omega-3s will also aid in general disease prevention, weight control (as long as you are not frying the fish), improved cognition, decreased stress, increased skin health, and an increased sense of well-being.

A quick note on diabetics, omega-3s, and heart disease. Researchers at the Harvard School of Public Health reported finding that women with diabetes who ate fish one to three times per month reduced their risk of coronary heart disease by 30%, while those who ate fish five or more times per week reduced their risk by more than 60%. See Chapter Three for recommended sources of seafood.

Perricone Recommendation: 1000 mg of fish oil three times per day, preferably with meals

SUPER CITRIMAX®

Two important strategies in AGE prevention are *calorie restriction (CR)* (more about this in Chapter Seven) and *reduction of body mass*. As we learned in our discussion of omega-3 EFAs, AGEs are now believed to be the cause of atherosclerosis, the leading cause of heart disease and stroke. Unfortunately, we are in an obesity epidemic the likes of which has never been seen before—and it is growing as fast as our waistlines; most people find it almost impossible to diet and avoid temptation in the face of so much (unhealthy and fattening) bounty. Fortunately, we have viable tools that can help us achieve these goals. One in particular, Super CitriMax, has had significant scientific testing, and the results have been extremely positive.

The Cell Plasma Membrane, EFAs, and AGE Formation

We need both omega-3 and omega-6 essential fatty acids (EFAs). Western diets have an overabundance of omega-6, which is dangerous because this surfeit is pro-inflammatory. On the other hand, we do not have enough omega-3s in our daily diets—bad news because these fats are anti-inflammatory. As we know, an important negative effect of AGE formation is the tremendous amount of disease-promoting inflammation they generate.

One of science's experts on essential fatty acids is Artemis P. Simopoulos, M.D. Dr. Simopoulos is a graduate of Barnard College, Columbia University, with a major in chemistry, and a graduate of the Boston University School of Medicine. Since 1984, Dr. Simopoulos's research focus has been on the evolutionary aspects of diet and the omega-6/omega-3 balance. Dr. Simopoulos has found several sources of information suggesting that human beings evolved on a diet with a ratio of omega-6 to omega-3 EFAs of approximately 1:1.

In today's Western diets the ratio is an amazing 15:1 to 16.7:1. That means that at least a whopping 15 times more omega-6s are ingested than omega-3s. This is also significantly out of step with the diet that we humans evolved and that established our genetic patterns—in fact after the dietary changes of the last 50 years it must be almost unrecognizable.

It's no wonder that we have an epidemic of depression and obesity, growing greater with each passing year. The simple truth is that these two conditions can be alleviated with omega-3 EFAs. Excessive amounts of omega-6 polyunsaturated fatty acids (PUFAs) and a very high omega-6/omega-3 ratio promote the pathogenesis of many diseases, including CVD, cancer, and inflammatory and autoimmune diseases, whereas increased levels of omega-3 PUFAs (a low omega-6/omega-3 ratio) exert suppressive effects. We need both, but must make sure that we have them in the proper proportions—which is no more than 5:1 omega-6s to omega-3s.

Say Goodbye to the Moody Blues

Super CitriMax helps increase levels of the "feel-good" hormone serotonin. Women in particular tend to crave high-glycemic carbohydrates to
raise their serotonin levels, which backfires. The carbs initially raise
these levels, but when our blood sugar drops, the serotonin goes with it,
leaving us feeling worse than before and encouraging us to reach for
another cookie.

The serotonin connection is an important one. Serotonin is a neurotransmitter found in the brain that affects both mood and appetite. Because
it is involved in the "satiety" action of Super CitriMax, it contributes the
following benefits:

- It reduces appetite, especially sugar and carbohydrate cravings.

- It improves spirits and promotes well-being, which can help prevent binge eating.

- It promotes restful sleep.

Ending the Constant Craving

Super CitriMax also combats cravings for sweet and starchy foods. These
two attributes alone are key strategies in fighting AGE formation—if we
don't feel depressed and we aren't craving carbs, we won't be contributing to AGE formation.

Super CitriMax is a patented, all-natural substance containing (−)-
hydroxycitric acid (HCA), an extract from the South Asian fruit *Garcinia
cambogia*, bound to the essential minerals calcium and potassium. The
dried *Garcinia cambogia* fruit has been used for centuries as a condiment
to make meals more filling. Super CitriMax has been clinically proven to
curb appetite, burn fat, and reduce body weight three times faster than
diet and exercise alone. It also blocks a key enzyme responsible for turning excess carbohydrates into fat and cholesterol. Importantly, Super
CitriMax works without affecting the central nervous system, and therefore will not cause side effects such as nervousness, rapid heart rate, or
insomnia.

Harry Preuss, M.D. and Debasis Bagchi, Ph.D., FACN, Adjunct Professor of Pharmacy at Creighton School of Pharmacy and Allied Health Professions, are two leading experts who have conducted clinical studies on Super CitriMax that have been published in peer-reviewed journals.

Super CitriMax is an extremely safe and effective product for weight control, and its claims are substantiated by numerous human clinical and preclinical studies—including gene studies—that have been published in peer-reviewed scientific journals. However, it is not intended to be a miracle diet cure; it is meant to be used as a complement to a healthy diet and exercise program. For our purposes, we can consider it an important ally in fighting obesity, body fat, metabolic syndrome, and the formation of AGEs.

SUPER CITRIMAX:

■ Reduces body weight three times faster than diet and exercise alone.

■ Increases serotonin (the feel-good hormone) while decreasing appetite.

■ Burns fat.

■ Inhibits fat production.

■ Lowers triglycerides, LDL, and total cholesterol (cardiovascular risk factors).

■ Increases beneficial HDL cholesterol.

■ Reduces body mass index (an indicator of healthy body weight).

Putting Fat in the Breakdown Lane

One great thing about Super CitriMax is that it does more than help you lose weight. Its positive effect on cholesterol levels is also very significant thanks to the inclusion of ChromeMate (see page 106).

A study conducted at Ohio State University Medical Center revealed yet another exciting finding. Using the fat tissue of overweight nondiabetic women, researchers discovered that Super CitriMax down-regulated (deactivated) a gene that helps preserve the protective perilipin protein layer surrounding aging fat cells. As fat cells age, the perilipin protein layer increases, which results in white fat turning into yellow fat and yellow fat turning into brown fat; the darker the fat, the more difficult it is to break it down. The study showed that Super CitriMax broke down the perilipin protein layer of more than 50% of the fat cells tested, resulting in the death of these cells and the release of fat metabolites, which helps with weight loss. This finding corroborates earlier studies showing that people who took Super CitriMax excreted higher levels of fat metabolites in their urine than people taking a placebo.

Perricone Recommendation: I recommend the Clinical Strength Super CitriMax, which also contains ChromeMate. The recommended dosage is 4500 milligrams, split into three doses of 1500 milligrams each, taken 30 minutes to 2 hours before meals.

RHODIOLA ROSEA

Both *Cinnamomi cassiae* (cinnamon) and *Rhodiola rosea* extracts have long histories as antidiabetic folk medicines. In Chapter Three you learned that cinnamon stimulates insulin receptors and inhibits an enzyme that inactivates these receptors, thereby increasing the cells' ability to use glucose. Thus, cinnamon may significantly help people with adult-onset diabetes normalize their blood-sugar levels.

Recent studies have shown that increased oxidative stress from free-radical damage plays a key role in both the cause and the development of diabetes and all its related complications, such as greatly accelerated AGE formation and related damage to all organ systems. This discovery again underscores the importance of targeted antioxidants in the prevention and treatment of degenerative diseases.

A study that particularly piqued my interest, "Antioxidative effects of *Cinnamomi cassiae* and *Rhodiola rosea* extracts in liver of diabetic mice," examined the effects of cinnamon and *Rhodiola rosea* extracts on blood sugar, lipid peroxidation (the breaking down of fats to form free radicals), glutathione levels, and the activity of antioxidants in the livers of mice. Researchers found that both cinnamon and *Rhodiola rosea* extracts significantly lowered blood sugar. At the same time, this combination increased levels of glutathione. As you have learned, glutathione levels decline with age, making us much more susceptible to disease. In combination, these two antioxidants also protected the destruction of fats from free-radical damage. In other words, they protected the good ones and decreased the bad ones. This is exciting news because we know that elevated glucose accelerates aging, disease, and AGE formation. Both cinnamon and *Rhodiola rosea* extracts are proving to be effective for correcting high blood sugar (hyperglycemia) and preventing diabetic complications.

As you learned earlier, glutathione is the most important antioxidant that our cells produce. It is critical in cells' defense against inflammation-generating free radicals and oxidative stress. Whenever cells are under severe oxidative stress, glutathione comes to the rescue. *Unfortunately, glutathione is rapidly used up. Therefore any substance that can increase its level is of tremendous importance in combating oxidative stress—a precipitator in many diseases, including diabetes. We need high levels of glutathione to protect our bodies from AGE-related damage.*

Additional studies with *Rhodiola rosea* found that it:

- Increased the ability to perform mental work even when fatigue and stress (key contributors to diminished mental capacity) are present;

- Is a safe and effective treatment for mild to moderate depression;

- Increased physical and mental endurance and performance.

Perricone recommendation: *Rhodiola rosea* root extract (standardized to 3% rosavins (7.5 mg), 1% salidrosides (2.5 mg), one 250-mg capsule daily

In the next chapter I introduce a new form of the dipeptide carnosine, which has remarkable antiglycating properties thanks to a revolutionary scientific breakthrough.

6.

The Carnosine Breakthrough

"Every second, a destructive process called 'glycation' occurs throughout the body. Glycation can be described as the binding of a protein molecule to a glucose molecule resulting in the formation of damaged, non-functioning structures. Many age-related diseases such as arterial stiffening, cataract and neurological impairment are at least partially attributable to glycation. The glycation process is presently irreversible."*

The quote above is from the experts at Life Extension Foundation, who succinctly state that "the glycation process is presently irreversible."

And they were right. Until now. The exciting news is that Perricone readers will be the first to learn about a significant breakthrough that now enables us to both prevent and reverse this glycation by adding a new form of carnosine to our armory of AGE protection.

CARNOSINE (B-ALANYL-L-HISTIDINE)

Carnosine is a naturally occurring dipeptide of the amino acids beta-alanine and histidine. It is often called a neuropeptide due to its brain-protective properties, and is highly concentrated in muscle and brain tissues and in the lenses of the eyes. Carnosine also occurs naturally in healthy muscles, and in the heart, brain, liver, kidneys, and other tissues. The muscles contain about 20 μmol/g dry weight. Carnosine—a superb antioxidant—prevents meat from going rancid. So the more carnosine contained in meat, the longer its shelf life.

Carnosine occurs naturally in the diet from high-protein foods such as meat (including poultry and fish). However, unless we are eating grass-fed beef (as opposed to grain-fed beef), our intake of beef should be limited to prevent eating too much saturated fat.

Many scientific studies have found that carnosine inhibits the formation of AGEs. Through its distinctive combination of antioxidant and antiglycating properties, it is able to decrease cellular oxidative stress, and it can reduce inflammation by inhibiting the formation of free radicals. By controlling oxidative stress, suppressing glycation, and chelating metal ions including copper, carnosine is able to reduce harmful damage to DNA. Studies have demonstrated that substances that inhibit glycation, including carnosine, work by binding copper in the body. Although we need small amounts of copper in our bodies, research shows that it can stimulate the formation of free radicals, inflammation, and glycation, resulting in AGEs.

Carnosine is also a very special kind of antioxidant. While many antioxidants act as anti-inflammatories to protect our cells from free radical damage, they cannot completely protect proteins from being damaged (misfolded). Carnosine is unique in that it can both repair and remove the misfolded proteins.

This misfolding of proteins is a normal cellular occurrence; however, if our nutrition, hygiene, or lifestyle is compromised, the misfolding is increased. Experts in protein function believe that the misfolding of proteins may account for as much as half of all human disease, either directly or indirectly (Alzheimer's and mad cow are just two of the most famous examples of diseases linked to protein damage). In the skin, these damaged proteins result in wrinkled, sagging skin and the loss of elasticity.

Carnosine inhibits glycation and cross-linking of proteins caused by aldehydes. Carnosine is effective in reducing AGE formation by competing with proteins for binding with sugars. As you will learn, carnosine acts as a "sacrificial" molecule, binding with the proteins and thereby preventing them from binding with the sugars—and thus stopping AGE formation.

How Carnosine Reverses AGEs

Carnosine is highly regarded as an antiglycating agent. Diseases that arise from AGE-related diabetic complications such as cataracts, neuropathy, arteriosclerosis, and kidney failure may be prevented or treated with carnosine. In fact, since AGEs affect everyone, although not as quickly or as debilitatingly as they do in diabetics, carnosine is a very important nutrient to both prevent AGE formation and to remove or repair AGE-damaged proteins.

A Case of Mistaken Identity

Here's how it works. Carnosine, being a small peptide, resembles a protein molecule. When carnosine gets near the linear or straight form of glucose (sugar) described in Chapter One, the sugar will bind or attach to the carnosine instead of the protein, thus "saving the life" of a nearby protein. Then that little carnosine with the sugar attached is taken out of the body via the kidneys. Very elegant. For that reason, carnosine is often called a "sacrificial" or "suicide" molecule. It saved the protein from becoming glycated by tricking the linear sugar molecule into thinking that it (the carnosine) was a protein molecule. Thus we can see how effective carnosine can be in its new modified and bioavailable form as an AGE-prevention strategy.

Carnosine also:

- buffers the effects of lactic acid in the muscles (the muscles' pH remains neutral even in heavy physical exercise, such as sport sprints);

- has many potent antioxidative actions;

- is able to inactivate reactive oxygen species and scavenge free radicals;

- can sequester aldehyde;

- prevents glycation;

- prevents carbonylation of proteins;

- functions as a neurotransmitter;

- bolsters proteasome pathways. (Proteasomes are protein-degradation "machines" within cells that digest a variety of proteins into short polypeptides and amino acids, thus helping dispose of damaged proteins); and

- chelates metals.

One of the negative side effects of aging is a decline in muscle mass, which may be related to declining carnosine levels. As we age, muscle mass decreases by more than 60%. Carnosine protects the cells in our muscles from free radical damage caused by exercise. It also helps the heart muscle function more efficiently.

Carnosine is also an *auto*regulator. This means that it is able to slow overactive body processes and increase underactive ones. For instance, carnosine can thin the blood of people whose blood tends to clot too much, and can increase clotting ability in those whose blood tends to clot inadequately. In those with overactive immune systems, carnosine can suppress the immune response. In those with weakened immune systems, such as older people or those in a poor state of health, carnosine can stimulate the immune response. Carnosine also normalizes brain-wave functions.

MCAR—THE NEW CARNOSINE

The carnosine that is currently available as a nutritional supplement is broken down or inactivated in the blood and other tissues. This occurs rapidly and is the work of a group of enzymes called dipeptidases or carnosinases.

In the past, people took high doses of carnosine to try to get a therapeutic effect. Unfortunately, this did not work, as the stomach and blood enzymes very quickly broke down the carnosine.

Working in a lab, a group of very progressive and brilliant biochemists has modified carnosine. By adding natural functional chemical groups to the carnosine molecule, they made it impervious to degeneration from the stomach and blood enzymes.

But that's not all. The scientists also attached other natural elements such as copper, zinc, magnesium, and manganese to carnosine to further enhance its efficacy. This complicated and highly creative process is not simply mixing minerals with carnosine and hoping for the best (the method of operation of many formulators). Instead it is the result of chemical reactions, in the laboratory setting, of the carnosine with the functional groups and minerals to form an entirely new molecule.

This new carnosine—called mCar—is dramatically different, and has no peer in the nutritional world. Without divulging patented proprietary trade secrets, suffice it to say that mCar significantly improves carnosine's absorption, allowing it to deliver up to 10 times more carnosine than the conventional form.

Benefits and properties of carnosine include the following.

- It extends life span 20% in senescence- (age)-accelerated mice.

  - It dramatically improves the behavior and appearance of old mice.

  - It preserves brain biochemical functions.

- It rejuvenates senescent (aging) human cells in culture.

  - It increases cell life span.

  - It restores youthful appearance and growth patterns in cells approaching senescence.

- It is the most effective natural glycation fighter.

  - It protects proteins from cross-linking.

  - It protects proteins from AGE toxicity.

  - It protects against formation of AGEs.

- It is a multifunctional protein protector.

  - It protects against formation of protein carbonyls, the hallmark of protein damage.

- It inhibits damaged proteins from damaging healthy proteins.

- It helps preserve normal protein turnover.

- It aids recycling of damaged proteins.

■ It protects against metal toxicity.

- It chelates copper and zinc, helping dissolve Alzheimer's disease plaques.

- It naturally protects against copper or zinc toxicity in the brain.

■ It is a versatile antioxidant and aldehyde scavenger.

- It protects against free-radical damage.

- It provides superior protection of chromosomes from oxygen damage.

■ It protects brain proteins and chemistry.

- It protects brain cells from excitotoxicity.

- It sharply reduces lipid peroxidation in brains of senescence-accelerated mice.

- It inhibits cross-linking of beta-amyloid into Alzheimer's disease plaques.

- It safeguards brain chemistry in rats that are overproducing free radical–induced inflammation.

DARA'S STORY

Dara is a former ballet dancer whose highly successful and visible career spanned several decades. Unfortunately, an injury on the tennis court brought her dancing to an abrupt end. However, she was still active behind the scenes when she and I met at fund-raiser dedicated to expanding school programs to include teaching the performing arts.

"Dr. Perricone, it is such a pleasure to meet you," she said as we were introduced. "I have been hoping our paths might cross one day," she added, clearly delighted that we would be seated next to each other at one of the elegantly set tables. Dara was a vivacious and entertaining dinner companion, and by the time the third course was served we felt like old friends. "Dr. Perricone, I hope you don't mind my asking you a professional question," she queried. "Not at all, Dara. Ask away," I answered.

"All of my life—since early childhood—I have been physically active, first in ballet school, which I started at the age of five, and then with sports, including tennis and swimming. Once I had that fall on the tennis court several years ago, I could no longer maintain the same level of intense activity, but I continue to exercise, just at a more leisurely pace. I still play tennis, but prefer doubles to singles, and I enjoy swimming on a regular basis."

She went on to explain that in the past couple of years she had noticed that her muscles were losing tone in her face, neck, and body. As a dancer, she was very aware of her musculature, perhaps more so than the average person, and what she was seeing was no figment of her imagination. She had gone through menopause in her very early 40s. Most women experience menopause between the ages of 40 and 55, so she was definitely on the early side of the equation. Smoking can also lead to early menopause, and like many dancers, she had been a smoker. Fortunately, she had given it up several years earlier.

Although testosterone is traditionally associated with males, women also have small amounts of this important hormone, which declines with menopause, as does another "youth" hormone, estrogen. The loss of these hormones results in physical changes to the body, such as loss of muscle mass, thickening in the waist, and thinning skin. Although Dara was thin, she had experienced weight gain in the abdominal area since menopause. However, it wasn't just the loss of muscle and the extra fat that were bothering her. She was also dismayed to find that her skin was looking wrinkled—and not just in the delicate eye area. She also observed lines on her upper lip, some of which can be attributed to her prior smoking habit, and on her forehead, cheeks, and throat.

While it was clear that Dara was experiencing the effects of menopause, including thinning skin and loss of muscle mass, these weren't caused only by menopause. Her skin and muscle damage could also be attributed to AGE formation. Although she was not addicted to sugar, like many women, she had made rice cakes a dietary staple to help keep her weight down. As you know, such snack foods raise blood sugar and insulin because they are rapidly broken down into simple sugars once eaten, thus promoting AGEs. Her smoking also accelerated AGEs, and both had conspired to make her look older than her years.

As a final insult, Dara was guilty of overexercising, which increases levels of the stress hormone cortisol. Cortisol is catabolic—that is, it breaks down muscle mass. In addition, cortisol has a direct impact on where in the body fat is deposited. Scientific studies have verified that cortisol promotes the storage of fat in the abdominal area. This meant that the weight Dara carried in her midsection, referred to as *central obesity*, is visceral fat, considered the most dangerous because it surrounds the vital organs. Visceral fat is metabolized by the liver, which turns it into blood cholesterol. Visceral fat also puts pressure on the heart and arteries, increasing the chances of heart trouble.

Menopause notwithstanding, one of the negative side effects of aging is the decline in muscle mass, which may be directly related to declining carnosine levels. In fact, as we age, muscle mass decreases by more than 60%. Exercise can be a double-edged sword in that it can keep us from being overweight, yet it can also create free-radical damage. The good news is that carnosine protects the cells in the muscles from this free-radical damage.

Dara's case gave me the perfect opportunity to work with mCar and put it to the test, both as a supplement and as a topical treatment. We set up a time to meet later that week in which I would outline a program for Dara. My greatest success has always been in combining diet, supplements, and topical treatments.

At our meeting we discussed Dara's food choices. She needed to avoid the rice cakes and replace them with foods rich in essential fats and antioxidants. Because we cannot store protein, we need to make sure that we have enough protein every day. I instructed her to have six ounces of protein at each meal. I recommended that she purchase a small kitchen scale and weigh her protein sources. The source should weigh six ounces before cooking. A good choice for a snack to replace the rice cakes was a small handful of nuts and an apple. I also gave her copies of food lists with recommended foods on one list and foods to avoid or enjoy in moderation on the other.

For supplements, in addition to a good multivitamin, Dara was instructed to take mCar, along with the antiglycating antioxidants alpha lipoic acid (ALA) and benfotiamine. In addition, I gave her conjugated linoleic acid (CLA) and niacin-bound chromium (NBC), both proven to decrease body fat and restore muscle mass. I also made sure that she took the omega-3 essential fatty acids—very important supplements—as well as astaxanthin and coenzyme Q-10, which are proven to help decrease skin wrinkling. These three nutrients occur at high levels in salmon, which is part of the reason salmon is such an anti-aging and wrinkle- and AGE-preventing food. However, even if Dara ate salmon several times per week, I wanted to make sure that she was getting additional amounts of these nutrients; hence the supplement recommendations. As a final important last step, I started her on a supplement known as branched-chain amino acids, consisting of leucine, isoleucine, and valine (see Resources section). This active group of amino acids is needed for the maintenance of muscle tissue, and appears to preserve muscle stores of glycogen (a stored form of carbohydrates that can be converted into energy).

For topical treatments, I gave Dara a special combination of topical antiglycating agents, including ALA and mCar. This unique form of carnosine has the amazing ability to actually reverse the signs of aging in old skin cells. It can restore the cells to their former more youthful appearance and also extend their life span. Carnosine's AGE-fighting powers are truly remarkable.

Dara and I made plans to meet in about eight weeks, to give her body time to adjust to the new regimen and accrue positive results. And accrue they did. As she approached, I could see from across the room that she had a new, dynamic radiance to her look. Up close it was even better. Dara's skin, which had appeared very fragile, had taken on a smooth suppleness. Gone was the papery, dry texture of eight short weeks earlier. Her face appeared plumper in all the right places, and the lines and wrinkles were significantly diminished. I have seen many people experience physical rejuvenation with the three-tiered program (diet, supplements, and topical treatments). However, I was particularly gratified to see the unmistakable effects of mCar on Dara's skin. I was just as gratified by what I didn't see. By rejuvenating the senescent skin cells, the carnosine had been able to stop age and AGE-related degeneration and visibly reverse the appearance of aging skin.

A NEW WAY TO PROTECT YOUR EYES

I recently had the opportunity to discuss the powerful eye-protecting effects of carnosine with Phil Micans, M.S., PharmB. I first met Phil in Monaco several years ago, when I was keynote speaker at the Monte Carlo Anti-aging Conference.

Phil is Vice President of International Aging Systems (IAS Group), the world's largest supplier of specialist medicine and nutrition. It is also a tremendous source of information about antiaging, preventive, and alternative medicine. IAS has also been at the forefront of disseminating a wealth of scientific studies and clinical information on protecting our eyes against the ravages of AGEs through the use of powerful antioxidants such as carnosine.

Vision Quest

AGEs are highly destructive to our eyes, and are responsible for cataract formation. Cataracts are the leading cause of blindness, accounting for about 42% of all cases of blindness worldwide—despite the availability of effective surgical treatment.

Today we have an appalling situation in which more than 17 million people worldwide are blind because of cataracts, and 28,000 new cases are reported every day. To make matters worse, developing countries lack surgeons trained to perform cataract operations.

In fact, it is becoming apparent that it will be impossible to eliminate the overall problems (including blindness) caused by cataracts using currently available procedures. And, even if there were enough trained physicians to perform the surgery, it is not without risk.

Cataract surgery is the most commonly performed surgical procedure in people over 65 years of age, and 43% of all visits to ophthalmologists by Medicare patients in the U.S. are directly associated with cataracts. While cataract surgery is generally recognized as one of the safest operations, there is a significant complication rate. For example, in the U.S., 30% to 50% of all patients having cataract extraction develop opacification (the process of becoming cloudy or opaque) of the posterior lens capsule within two years and require further laser treatment.

Since the number of cataract operations is so large, even a small percentage of complications represents a significant number of people. Of patients having cataract surgery, 0.8% later have retinal detachments, 0.6% to 1.3% are later hospitalized for corneal edema (or require corneal transplantation), and 0.1% present later with endophthalmitis (inflammation of the eye's interior). Thus, aside from secondary cataracts, about 2% of the 1.35 million (or approximately 27,000 individuals), *just in the U.S. each year,* develop serious complications as a result of cataract surgery.

Meanwhile, approximately 25% of the population over 65 (and about 50% over 80) have a serious loss of vision due to cataracts. Since this is the population most susceptible to lens opacification, and since this section of the population is expected to increase dramatically rather soon, the number of individuals with cataracts is set to reach epidemic proportions.

During cataract surgery, an eye doctor (ophthalmologist) removes the clouded lens from the eye and generally replaces the lens with an artificial lens. However, aside from any possible complications, an artificial lens simply does not have the overall optical qualities of a natural lens.

Thanks to some very important new cutting-edge research, we may now be able to safely treat existing cataracts and also prevent cataracts from forming in the first place.

Over the past several years, research from the East, particularly Russia, has focused on a special analogue of the dipeptide carnosine. This particular form is known as N-acetylcarnosine (NAC), and it has been proven highly effective in the treatment of cataracts. In fact, NAC presents the first major leap forward in the treatment and possible prevention of senile cataract.

Formulated into eyedrops, NAC provides treatment without surgery. This allows the patient to keep their natural lens rather than cope with an artificial one.

Human trials using NAC eyedrops, known as Can-C Eye Drops (see Resources section), applied twice daily in the eye for six months in patients suffering from senile cataract had the following results:

1. 88.9% had improvement of glare sensitivity.

2. 41.5% had improvement of the transmissivity of the lens (the lens was able to receive clear images).

3. 90% had improvement in visual acuity.

How NAC Works in the Eye

A cataract is a glycation problem. The proteins have become cross-linked (and hence impaired). The result of this reaction leads to the discoloration of the eye-lens to yellow and brown, impairing the vision. The lens becomes hardened and discolored due to lifelong AGE cross-linking of the lens proteins. This persists in the aqueous humor (the clear, watery fluid circulating in the chamber of the eye between the cornea and the lens). This is the result of the low availability of natural defenses in the form of antioxidants, which decline with advancing age.

Carnosine is known to compete on the molecule for the glycating agent and to protect cellular structures against aldehydes. Therefore, carnosine can help prevent proteins from becoming cross-linked and slow the cross-linking process (and in this case prevent the proteins from becoming cataracts).

NAC has also been shown to be highly resistant to *carnosinase*, the natural enzyme that breaks L-carnosine down. NAC delivers L-carnosine into the aqueous humor of the eye, where it acts as a natural and comprehensive antioxidant, protecting structural lens proteins from the free radical–induced oxidation process.

L-carnosine is an excellent antioxidant, and is particularly effective against potent free radicals, especially the superoxide and hydroxyl forms of free radicals. It is therefore presumed that the antioxidant role of L-carnosine within the aqueous humor is a major factor in preventing cataracts and slowing their progression.

However, when L-carnosine eyedrops were used, there was *no* presence of L-carnosine in the aqueous humor, even after 30 minutes. This may be because L-carnosine is broken down before it reaches the aqueous humor. So, NAC may act as a "carrier" for L-carnosine, delivering it where it is needed.

The powerful antioxidant abilities of carnosine within the eye, and the prevention of cross-linking, help explain why NAC is effective at preventing cataracts, slowing their progression, and perhaps even halting them. This doesn't explain why NAC has been shown to reverse cataracts. However, we may already know the answer.

When carnosine is delivered in high doses, it can reverse the protein-aldehyde cross-linking described earlier in this chapter (this reaction is normally very difficult to reverse) and has been shown to have a "rejuvenating" effect on cultured cells.

The NAC Benefit

We may logically ask why NAC eyedrops have been shown to have this action upon cataracts while L-carnosine (which is its sister dipeptide) appears to have little benefit. Dr. Mark Babizhayev, one of the principal Russian researchers behind the clinical trials with NAC eyedrops, gave us this reply.

"I believe that the application of L-carnosine for the treatment of human cataracts is misleading. This is because L-carnosine readily becomes a substrate for the activity of natural peptidases (i.e., carnosinase) in the aqueous humor. So much so that there is *no* sign of L-carnosine in the aqueous humor within 15 minutes after instillation. Furthermore, I consider that L-carnosine eyedrops may even be harmful for eyes because they gradually release histamine, which, located as it would be in the presence of the eye lens, is a very toxic agent. However, NAC eyedrops are resistant to hydrolysis with natural carnosinase. Therefore, NAC is the only currently known agent that reverses and prevents human cataracts."

In the case of eyedrops, L-carnosine *must* be avoided—use only eyedrops containing NAC (labeled CAN-C Eye Drops).

NAC eyedrops have been shown to have measurable effects within only one month of use. However, it is recommended that for maximum efficacy one should continue using them for at least 3 to 5 months. In addition, the drops' effectiveness is increased the sooner they are used after a cataract is detected. Also, considering that senile cataracts are an ongoing aging disorder, NAC eyedrops may be required on a regular basis to help maintain the eye's natural antioxidant defenses.

Additional Benefits

Other than senile cataracts, NAC may have other benefits. Although the information is not yet published, the unique NAC formula of CAN-C Eye Drops, with its added and synergistic lubricants, may also provide beneficial results with the following eye disorders:

- Presbyopia (the gradual loss of the eye's ability to change focus from far away to close. This occurs in almost everyone sometime after the age of 40)

- Open-angle primary glaucoma (in combination with beta-blockers)

- Corneal disorders

- Computer vision syndrome

- Eye strain

- Ocular inflammation

- Blurred vision

- Dry eye syndrome

- Retinal diseases

- Vitreous opacities and lesions

- Complications of diabetes mellitus and other systemic diseases

- Contact lens difficulties, particularly with soft contact lenses. (Not only do the lubricants in the Can-C Eye Drops help make wearing contact lenses more comfortable, but they are also believed to reduce the buildup of lactic acid in the eye, thus enabling the lens to be left safely in the eye for a longer period of time).

The Clear-Sighted Results

A July 2000 study at China's Harbin Medical University found the following results with NAC eyedrops. NAC eyedrops were used in a clinical trial to treat 96 patients aged 60 and above. All the patients had senile cataracts in various degrees of maturity. The duration of the disease in these patients ranged between 2 and 21 years.

First, the researchers stopped the patients' use of all other anticataract drugs. Then the patients instilled 1 or 2 drops into each eye 3 or 4 times a day, for a period of 3 to 6 months.

The level of eyesight improvement and the change of lens transparency were considered evaluation indexes. The results showed that there was a pronounced effect on *primary senile cataract;* the effective rate was 100% (i.e., all patients experienced an improvement). For the more *mature senile cataract* (i.e., those who had had the cataract the longest time, in some cases more than 20 years) the effective rate was still an extremely impressive 80%.

These are remarkable results considering that the best that could normally be expected would be a slight improvement and/or a halt to the progression, or under nontreated circumstances, a continual worsening of the disease.

It is also important to note that no side effects were seen in any of the patients.

Another Russian study was designed to document and quantify the changes in lens clarity over a 6- to 24-month period for 49 volunteers. Their average age was 65, and all suffered from senile cataracts with minimal to advanced opacification.

Patients received either a 1% solution of NAC eyedrops or a placebo, 2 drops twice a day into each eye. They were then evaluated at 2- and 6-month periods. The tests consisted of ophthalmoscopy (glare test), a stereocinematographic test (split-image test), and retro-illumination (photography). A computerized digital analysis then displayed the light-scattering and absorbing effects of the centers of each lens.

At 6 months, 88.9% of all eyes treated with NAC had an improvement in glare sensitivity (the lowest individual score was a 27% improvement;

the highest was 100% improvement). Of all eyes treated with NAC, 41.5% had a significant improvement in the *transmissivity* of the lens. But perhaps most important, 90% of the eyes treated with NAC showed an improvement in visual acuity. Meanwhile, in the placebo group there was little change in eye quality at 6 months and a gradual deterioration at 12 to 24 months.

This study also showed that at 24 months the NAC-treated group (which already had significant improvement in the quality of their eyesight) sustained these results with continued use of the NAC eyedrops.

Once again, no significant side effects were noted in any cases throughout the 2-year period.

Not Just for Cataracts

Another interesting study evaluated patients between the ages of 48 and 60 who had various degrees of eyesight impairment, but who did *not* have symptoms of cataracts. After a course of treatment ranging from 2 to 6 months, the conclusion was that the eyedrops alleviated eye tiredness and continued to improve eyesight (i.e., there was more clear vision). The subjects reported that the treatment "brightened" and "relaxed" their eyes. This is an important indicator that the eyedrops have a value for both preventive purposes and medical applications.

IN CONCLUSION

We know that cataracts develop when antioxidant defense is exhausted, leading to the cross-linking of the lens *crystallins*, producing a clouded lens, and hence impaired eyesight, that is eyesight that is diminished in strength quality or utility. Therefore we can comfortably assume that the regular use of a 1% NAC eyedrop (as used in the clinical trials) delivers "a high dose of carnosine capable of reversing the lens cross-linking," and hence capable of the reduction and eradication of cataracts.

NAC eyedrops appear to act as a universal antioxidant, both in the lipid (fat) phase of the cellular lens membranes and in the aqueous (water) environment. NAC eyedrops reduce and protect the crystalline lens from oxidative stress–induced, cross-linking damage.

Cataracts are a widespread age-related affliction, and NAC eyedrops appear to be a highly efficacious and safe treatment for them. As such, I suspect that this supplement is going to become one of the most important new discoveries, and will have a major impact on the way that cataracts are controlled.

Even if the development of cataracts can be delayed by 10 years, the overall benefits will be highly significant both from an individual's health and mobility viewpoint and because of the decreased burden placed on health-care providers.

Perricone recommended dosage: one to two drops in each eye twice per day or as directed by your physician. To order or to learn more about CAN-C Eye Drops, visit www.antiaging-systems.com

---

* Opening quote and summary reprinted with permission from "Why Antioxidants Aren't Enough," *Life Extension*, January 2002.

7.

The Newest Anti-Glycating Agents: CoQ-10, Glutathione, Pyridoxamine, Pycnogenol®, and Resveratrol

I n the course of writing this book, I have had the great good fortune to collaborate with some of the world's most forward-thinking scientists and biochemists, whose remarkable breakthroughs with stem-cell therapy, carnosine, glutathione, and CoQ-10 are destined to positively impact the lives of millions of people worldwide.

In Chapter Six you learned about a major breakthrough in the modification of the carnosine molecule, making it totally bioavailable to the body. Its superior antiglycating abilities enable us to rejuvenate the body both inside and out by preventing AGE formation and also by repairing and removing AGE-damaged proteins.

However, this is not the only exciting breakthrough we have to report. These same biochemists have modified both glutathione and coenzyme Q-10 (CoQ-10), and, as you will learn, these modifications will have far-reaching beneficial effects in preventing and treating AGEs and the inflammatory diseases they cause.

COQ-10: POWERFUL TOOL

CoQ-10 is naturally present in small amounts in a wide variety of foods, particularly in organ meats such as heart, liver, and kidney, as well as beef, soy oil, sardines, mackerel, and peanuts. However, it is important to supplement this key nutrient for the purposes of mitochondrial protection, rejuvenation, repair, and anti-aging. For optimal absorption into the bloodstream, CoQ-10 should be taken with foods that contain healthy fats, such as nuts and seeds, a salad dressed with extra-virgin olive oil, a piece of grilled salmon, or avocado slices.

CoQ-10, also called ubiquinone, is a fat-soluble vitamin-like substance present in every cell of the body. It is a powerful antioxidant/anti-inflammatory with many benefits, including its ability to increase energy production in the cell, treat and prevent obesity, and prevent many of the negative effects of AGEs.

CoQ-10 is well known for its ability to protect all the vital organs of the body, including the brain, heart, and kidneys. It keeps the heart muscle strong and healthy, and prevents the artery inflammation that leads to arteriosclerosis. Arteriosclerosis is a form of atherosclerosis, and as you learned in Chapter Five, AGEs are the major cause of atherosclerosis, which in turn is at the very root of heart disease.

CoQ-10 also maximizes the burning of foods for fuel, helping normalize fats in our blood. As you have learned, excess lipids and cholesterol in the blood can result in cardiovascular disease. As cells age, their energy production decreases. This means that their ability to repair themselves also decreases. Working synergistically with nutrients such as alpha lipoic acid in the energy-producing portion of cells known as the mitochondria, CoQ-10 enhances the cells' metabolism, giving us greater energy and endurance, and thereby preventing the aging cells' energy decline.

CoQ-10 also works synergistically with other antioxidants to elevate cellular levels of vitamins C and E and glutathione, and to help regulate blood sugar and enhance insulin sensitivity—powerful AGE-preventive benefits.

CoQ-10 Breakthrough in Diabetes and AGEs

Throughout this book I have discussed the damage caused by diabetes, a disease characterized by accelerated AGE formation, and how it wreaks havoc in all organ systems. It should come as no surprise that many of the complications arising from diabetes, often termed the "sugar" disease, stem from the sugar bonds of glycation. Therefore, to stop AGE formation we need to look at the many therapeutic interventions designed to prevent and treat diabetes.

As you have already learned, diabetes has become a much more common disease over the decades. Type 1 diabetes, a very serious disease, is caused by the total failure of the pancreas to produce insulin. Many people are under the mistaken impression that because insulin is readily available to people who need it, the disease is no longer the ominous threat that it used to be. However, without treatment, severe health consequences, usually ending in early death, are inevitable. But after decades of following patients with type 1 diabetes on insulin therapy, we now know that there are numerous negative consequences even for patients who are being treated daily with insulin injections.

In addition, type 2 diabetes, once known as adult-onset diabetes, is now becoming a much more widespread problem. In fact, there is a much higher incidence of this disease in both adults and children. Type 2 diabetes is characterized by a functioning pancreas (i.e., one with the ability to produce insulin). However, there is significantly diminished sensitivity to insulin in peripheral (external) tissue. This essentially means that the pancreas is excreting insulin, yet blood sugar continues to rise, due to the fact that the cells have become insensitive to the circulating insulin, and glucose cannot get into the cells.

Scientists and clinical physicians have spent years researching causes of, therapies for, and clinical changes in diabetes. This vast quantity of knowledge has been beneficial in making advances in fighting this unfortunately all-too-common disease.

As an anti-aging researcher, I have personally found the available information extremely useful because diabetes is the perfect model for accelerated aging. This means that the changes that occur in diabetics in a few years are equal to the changes that are seen in decades in nondiabetic adults. This is particularly true when it comes to the formation of AGEs and related damage.

We now know that elevated circulating glucose leads to accelerated glycation of tissue and chronically elevated levels of inflammation, resulting in an excess of blood fats (hyperlipidemia) and elevated cholesterols (hypercholesterolemia)—two conditions that lead to atherosclerosis and heart disease.

The negative effects of glucose (sugar) resulting in glycation are the core of this book. To aid us in the battle against AGE formation in nondiabetic aging, we need to take a strong look at the effects of various therapeutic interventions used on diabetics and extrapolate that information for AGE prevention and treatment, using new strategies that are not pharmacological but are instead natural nutrients.

What the Studies Show

Remember this key fact: High blood sugar generates free radicals, resulting in protein glycation, thereby causing damage to the normal enzyme systems that protect us from free radicals. And it is these free radicals that are responsible for many of the complications of diabetes. We can see that both diabetes and AGEs increase oxidative stress throughout the body. Powerful antioxidant therapies such as CoQ-10 can be of tremendous benefit to those at risk.

It is interesting to note that physicians studying the myriad physiological changes seen in diabetes' complicated disease process rely on animal models for many of their studies. Since diabetic animals are not readily found in nature, scientists need to induce diabetes by the use of a medication known as streptozotocin, which renders the pancreas nonfunctional.

One of the most exciting recent findings in streptozotocin-induced diabetic rats is the use of a new form of CoQ-10 to prevent the many detrimental changes caused by diabetes. Some of the changes seen were very similar to the changes that humans with diabetes experience, including elevated cholesterol and triglyceride levels, increased oxidation of fats (lipid peroxidation), and a decrease in good cholesterol (high-density lipoproteins, or HDL).

In fact, scientists were surprised to discover that CoQ-10 produced a decrease in blood-sugar levels even though insulin levels were already extremely low. They also found that, in addition to a decrease in serum cholesterol and tryglycerides, there was an increase in HDL, which is protective against heart disease. And there was a reduction in lipid peroxidation, meaning that lower levels of pro-inflammatory chemicals are circulating in these animals—which, as we have discussed repeatedly, decreases the risk of *all* disease processes.

Another unexpected benefit seen was the decrease in the elevated blood pressure that is usually seen in diabetic rats. All the negative changes that were seen in the diabetic rats, and that are also present in humans, can be treated with CoQ-10. This remarkable nutrient can reduce both AGE-related and the diabetes-induced complications that are so threatening to the brain and the body.

The Good Gets Better

Research scientists have worked their magic on CoQ-10 to create a highly absorbable new form of this important nutrient. This form of CoQ-10 is more bioavailable than any other CoQ-10 or ubiquinol available on the market today. Perricone recommended dosage: 30 mg per day. This CoQ-10:

- is 18 times more bioavailable in humans than ordinary CoQ-10;
- is absorbed in a standardized intestinal cell several times better than other brands of CoQ-10;
- is one of the most potent anti-aging compounds that can be marketed in the U.S.;
- lowers creatinine, a waste product from protein in the diet and from the muscles of the body, in urine levels in a human study, indicating that it blocks protein oxidation in the human body (The amount of creatinine in blood and urine can show whether the kidney is functioning properly.);

■ is one of the few compounds ever proven to lower DNA damage rates in humans, a difficult and rare accomplishment; lowering DNA damage rates more than 50% has enormous anti-aging and life span–increasing potential in humans; and

■ dissolves rapidly in water, is highly stable, and has no taste.

CoQ-10 is also blazing a very important trail in wrinkle prevention. But before you race to your local drugstore to stock up on the over-the-counter CoQ-10 creams and lotions, read on. Scientists have discovered that when it comes to fighting wrinkles, an oral CoQ-10 supplement may be the best way to go.

LAUREL'S STORY

I first met Laurel at the opening of one of her solo shows at an art gallery in midtown Manhattan. She is a very talented artist whose oil pastels of the hills of Tuscany are among some of my favorites in the contemporary art world.

Laurel is a tall and striking brunette in her mid 40s. As I made arrangements to return after the show to pick up my new painting, I congratulated her on the success of her opening.

"I knew I recognized you," she said with a happy smile. "Would it be possible for me to schedule an appointment for a professional consultation?" I gave her my business card and told her to call the office to arrange a time and date.

Several weeks later, Laurel arrived for her scheduled appointment. As we discussed her concerns, it soon became apparent that her biggest worry was the appearance of her skin. She believed that the last few years of career stress were accelerating the aging in her face. The huge interest generated in her work had meant that she had had to work almost round the clock to meet the demands of her many galleries. She was at the point of exhaustion, but knowing how ephemeral fame can be, she felt obliged to meet all of her many commitments.

I could see that she looked somewhat haggard. Therefore I did not doubt that she needed a good long rest. Since that was out of the question, the next-best strategy was to help her to increase her stamina and energy levels through improved nutrition and targeted supplements. This would benefit her physically as well as help restore her skin to a healthier state.

Fortunately, I had been working with a new and exciting proprietary blend of nutrients that were showing remarkable effectiveness at dramatically decreasing wrinkles while increasing skin elasticity—and not just the *appearance* of the wrinkles. This oral wrinkle reducer permanently shrinks them. Laurel was the ideal candidate for this new supplement.

Laurel's skin was dry, and she had sun damage, enlarged pores, the aforementioned wrinkles, and a loss of elasticity in her face and neck. I was eager to get her started.

An Inside Job

As you have learned in this book, many of the problems of aging and aging skin are caused by internal conditions, particularly AGE formation, which was apparent in Laurel's situation. AGEs are key mediators in inhibiting the growth of skin cells; in fact, AGEs slow or block the growth process. Although not a sun worshipper, Laurel was an avid gardener, and she had accrued quite a bit of sun damage. Unfortunately, AGE-damaged skin experiences much greater harm from the free radicals generated by sun exposure than do cells that have not been debilitated by AGE formation. In fact, once the proteins in the skin have become glycated, the skin is at an increased risk for both accelerated aging and skin cancer. To this end, I have created an oral antiwrinkle treatment that helps combat the effects of AGEs both internally and externally. In this way we can get to the very basis of the problems caused by aging, sun exposure, and AGEs. Since AGEs are an internal problem, it makes a lot of sense to have an internal solution as well as a topical one. In this way we can approach the problems from all angles, assuring us of a greater resolution.

A scientific study on key ingredients in my Total Skin and Body Supplements containing the oral wrinkle-reducing formula found significant changes in the study subjects. These included a decrease in the number of skin wrinkles and an increase in the skin's elasticity and moisture content. There was also an improvement in the skin's condition, which was described by the researchers as a change from rough skin to fresh and youthful skin.

How this synergistic mix of supplements may work to reduce wrinkles was addressed in another human study, in which the researchers found that the supplements' powerful antioxidant properties actually prevented DNA damage. DNA damage is believed to be one of the biggest factors (if not the biggest factor) responsible for both cancer and aging. To put this DNA damage prevention to the test, the supplements were given to smokers over a six-week period at the same low (30-mg) dose used in the wrinkle-reduction study.

Smokers were chosen because it is well known from earlier studies that smokers have higher whole-body DNA damage rates than nonsmokers, and that AGEs are a significant contributing factor to these rates.

After just six weeks, the whole-body DNA damage rate of the smokers taking the supplements was reduced by a whopping 51%. Decreasing a person's DNA damage rate by more than 50% holds enormous potential for slowing the aging process and preventing the diseases associated with aging. Remember this important fact: Glycation and AGEs attack not only the proteins in the body, but also the fats and the DNA, making these discoveries extremely important in our quest for AGE prevention and reversal of its damage.

These are amazing results from one product: reducing skin wrinkles and potentially living longer by cutting your DNA damage rate in half.

Other ingredients included in the oral wrinkle-reducing formula include:

Hyaluronic acid: Hyaluronic acid is a major component of connective tissue found mainly in the skin. Hyaluronic acid's primary function in the body is to bind water to connective tissues to keep them hydrated. Unfortunately, as with so many good things, the levels of this critical nutrient decline greatly with age—by the time we reach the age of 50, our bodies are producing about 50% less than they did in our youth. And it is believed that this decline is a major contributing factor to both joint ailments such as arthritis and wrinkled, sagging skin.

When used in topical products, hyaluronic acid has been found to be a potent wrinkle reducer. It is often used in conjunction with vitamin C, as it helps the vitamin to be absorbed into the skin, increasing its effectiveness.

Carotenes: One of the reasons I have always been such an advocate of eating salmon is that it possesses the carotenoid *astaxanthin* (it also contains wrinkle fighters CoQ-10 and omega-3 essential fatty acids). This member of the carotene family is responsible for the deep red or pink color of the salmon, and it has many wrinkle-fighting benefits, as does the entire carotenoid family. When taken as a dietary supplement, astaxanthin has been proven to provide powerful protection against photoaging, protecting the skin from the aging and damaging effects of the sun. Studies have also shown that supplemental astaxanthin supports even skin tone, significantly reduces wrinkles, and improves skin's elasticity. Astaxanthin is a critical strategy in combating both the internal and the external effects of aging and AGEs.

This new wrinkle-reducing formula also contains a broad spectrum of other carotenes. These carotenes are concentrated from a very special form of palm oil that contains the richest, most complete blend of all the carotenes in the world. The list of carotenes is comprehensive, and includes alpha-carotene, beta-carotene, lycopene, zeaxanthin, lutein, and beta-cryptoxanthin.

Numerous scientific studies show that oral supplementation with carotenes, especially lycopene and beta-carotene, improve skin structure, have powerful wound-healing properties, and offer great protection from damage caused by sunlight. In addition to their skin-rejuvenating and -protective properties, the carotenes lutein and zeaxanthin also protect against eye degeneration caused by sunlight, and other factors such as aging. As you have learned, AGEs attack the proteins in all organ systems, and are extremely damaging to both the skin and the eyes.

Vitamin C: I have been working for decades with vitamin C because it is one of the most powerful known stimulators of collagen production in the human skin. However, vitamin C levels in skin decline dramatically with age, resulting in a drop in collagen levels, and placing us at increased risk of damage from the sun's rays.

Collagen is the protein that provides and maintains the healthy, firm structure of human skin. Collagen prevents wrinkles and the saggy, baggy, droopy look seen in many older people's faces. As you have learned, collagen is one of the proteins attacked by circulating sugars, resulting in glycation and AGE formation. Vitamin C is important both topically (applied to the skin in its fat-soluble form) and also when taken as an oral supplement; in this form it can significantly increase collagen synthesis.

As a powerful water-soluble antioxidant, vitamin C quenches the oxygen species produced from sunlight exposure, and protects the body against the internal aging process. The effect of dietary vitamin C in the body is one more illustration of the fact that the appearance of our skin is a mirror of own internal body chemistry. Deep wrinkles and sagging skin are connected to glycosylated proteins in the collagen. This AGE-degraded collagen is not only visible in the skin, it also clearly reflects similar disasters affecting the internal organs. This is why we need to address the problem both internally and externally.

Tocotrienols: Natural vitamin E contains four chemically related compounds called *tocotrienols.* Tocotrienols are a form of "super" vitamin E, and I have been using them for many years, as both a supplement and in topical formulations. Tocotrienols are up to 40 times more potent than vitamin E itself in protecting the body against damage from sunlight, the aging process, and free radicals. Concentrations of alpha tocotrienol levels in the skin are many times higher than that of vitamin E itself. The wrinkle-reducing formula contains alpha tocotrienol along with the other naturally occurring tocotrienols to slow the aging process of the skin and to protect the skin from sun damage.

Pycnogenols: Studies have found that the antioxidant pycnogenol® acts as a collagen stabilizer by binding to collagen in the skin and maintaining elasticity, saving it from destruction. This action helps keep the skin firm and prevents wrinkles. Pycnogenol also improves microcirculation of tiny skin capillaries, which help support better oxygen, nutrient, and hydration supplies to the skin.

These substances that offer protection to the skin when taken internally are especially important in light of the current discussions on the efficacy and safety of many topical sunscreens.

To help with Laurel's enlarged pores, uneven skin tone, loss of radiance, lines, and wrinkles, I gave her a topical antiglycation formula that contained mCar, alpha lipoic acid, and other very powerful antioxidants. As a dermatologist, I admit to having a particular fondness for topical formulas with a great deal of efficacy, and I was also very interested in how the formula and the topical products would complement each other.

Putting It to the Test

Laurel was eager to get started on the Total Skin and Body supplements and the topicals, and was particularly delighted to learn that scientific studies promised visible and measurable results in as little as six weeks.

As luck would have it, we did not have our follow-up appointment until almost eight weeks later due to conflicting schedules. However, the timing could not have been better. Laurel's exhibition had ended, and she was able to deliver my new painting in person.

I could see great change in her skin. The many deep lines and webs of wrinkles were significantly reduced. But what most impressed me was the freshness of her complexion. It had a radiant look, and her skin had taken on a new softness. In addition, renewed elasticity was evident in a firmer, suppler appearance. This was the effect of the renewed collagen production. Her gray pallor had been replaced with a healthy glow, the hallmark of young skin. And her skin was now well hydrated, with the plumped-up appearance of increased moisture content.

The alpha lipoic acid (ALA) in the topical formula had also increased the flow of nitric acid to Laurel's skin, resulting in increased blood circulation and much healthier coloring. It had also greatly reduced pore size and dryness, thanks to its powerful anti-inflammatory properties. ALA is superb as an antiglycating agent, and when combined with mCar it dramatically decreases the cross-hatching type of lines and wrinkles that herald AGE damage. All in all, the transformation was quite radical and exciting.

"I have to say, Dr. Perricone, that when I look in the mirror, I feel like I am seeing the picture of Dorian Gray in reverse," Laurel laughed. Truth be told, I couldn't have agreed with her more. To learn more about the oral wrinkle-reducing Total Skin Body formula, see the Resources section.

GLUTATHIONE

As you learned in Chapter Five, glutathione (GSH) is a powerful water-soluble antioxidant found in all cells of our body. GSH is a tripeptide; that is, it consists of three amino acids: cysteine, glycine, and glutamic acid. It is important in cellular respiration, the process in which a cell breaks down sugar or other organic compounds to release energy used for cellular work.

GSH is the most important antioxidant our cells produce. It is critical in cells' defense against AGE-mediated inflammation-generating free radicals and oxidative stress. Whenever a cell is under severe oxidative stress, glutathione comes to the rescue. To understand how important this is, consider this fact: Glutathione is so effective in preventing inflammation in the body that it is being used to treat people who suffer from the high levels of inflammation and body wasting resulting from HIV infection.

However, GSH is quickly depleted, and levels drop rapidly. Low GSH levels are seen in virtually every inflammatory state, and are almost perfect indicators of chronic and acute inflammatory states.

GSH is also an important detoxifying agent, enabling the body to eliminate toxins and poisons. It also regulates and regenerates our immune cells. And it protects enzyme proteins that inhibit collagen-digesting enzymes. These enzymes cause damage to the skin, leading to wrinkles, or scars in the area of acne lesions.

It is almost impossible to overstate GSH's importance as the body's primary antioxidant defense system. It is required for the smooth functioning of all cells. It is involved in protein synthesis, amino acid transport, and the recycling of other antioxidants, such as vitamins C and E and CoQ-10, assisting their function in protecting the cell. Alpha lipoic acid (ALA), which we discussed in Chapter Five, also works synergistically with other antioxidants to raise levels of vitamins C and E, CoQ-10, and GSH in the cell. Each of these nutrients is critical in helping protect the body from glycation.

Network Antioxidants

According to Dr. Lester Packer, a well-known pioneer in antioxidants, until recently, each antioxidant was thought to work independently of the others. We know now that that's not true. The antioxidants all work together like musicians in a symphony. Dr. Packer has labeled some of them "network antioxidants." What makes network antioxidants special is that they can greatly enhance one another's power.

Dr. Packer notes that "Although there are literally hundreds of antioxidants, only five appear to be network antioxidants: Vitamins C and E, glutathione, lipoic acid, and CoQ-10. Vitamins C and E are not produced in the body but must be obtained through food. Glutathione, lipoic acid, and CoQ-10 are produced by the body, but levels of these antioxidants decline as we age. That is why we need to supplement all of them."

However, until now, GSH supplementation was not a viable reality, because supplemental GSH is rapidly digested in the gastrointestinal system, destroying the supplement's activity. N-acetylcysteine and ALA, precursors or building blocks of GSH, can be taken orally, as these substances work synergistically to elevate levels of GSH in the cell. But now we have a better way—more about this on page 155.

Network Antioxidants in Action

As discussed previously, when free radicals attack the cell plasma membrane (the outer portion of the cell), they tend to oxidize fats and activate enzymes, resulting in a tidal wave of pro-inflammatory chemicals flowing into the cell. To compound the problem, the inflammation produced triggers the production of more free radicals. Once an inflammatory cascade has begun, GSH is quickly depleted, leading to even greater inflammation. To prevent the destructive effects of inflammation caused by free radicals, powerful antioxidants such as GSH enable other antioxidants and anti-inflammatories, such as vitamins C and E, to effectively protect all portions of the cell, both the fat-soluble cell plasma membrane and the water-soluble portion of the cell known as the cytosol.

When scientists want to see who's winning the fight between free radicals and antioxidants, they look at the balance between the two. This balance is known as the "redox" status of the cell, the ratio of oxidants (bad guys) to reducing agents or antioxidants (good guys). If cells don't maintain the correct redox status, pro-inflammatory chemicals are created. When they are released they cause severe damage on all levels, leading to virtually every disease process we can think of, from acne and Alzheimer's to diabetes and cancer.

Remember that AGEs change GSH redox status and that GSH plays an essential role in maintaining redox status in the cell. AGEs are cytotoxic;

Long Live the Insects!

Interestingly, it isn't just humans who respond to GSH. Plants also produce it, and when they are injured, they produce more of it. Studies have shown that insects will preferentially feed on injured plants. When insects are getting this extra GSH, they become larger. Other studies have shown that boosting tissue levels of GSH in mosquitoes causes them to live 40% longer.

that is, they are deadly to the cell. We must have adequate GSH in all our cells to regulate the redox status and block the inflammation, AGE formation, and damage.

Published clinical and scientific research has demonstrated that GSH:

- is a potent antiviral against human herpes simplex virus (HSV-1), while leaving normal cells healthy;

- selectively targets and kills cancer lymphoma cells, while leaving normal cells healthy;

- selectively targets and kills other malignant cancer cells;

- ameliorates inflammation;

- neutralizes free radicals and prevents free radical formation;

- stimulates anti-aging enzymes in human cells;

- is the strongest anticancer agent manufactured by the human body;

- relieves arthritis symptoms;

- relieves Parkinson's symptoms;

- enhances weight/mass increase to sustain the immune-response system in cachetic patients (those suffering from extreme weight loss);

- protects against damage from smoking and air pollution;

- minimizes and controls asthma;

- protects against radiation damage;

- repairs liver damage caused by alcohol and hepatitis;

- refreshes spent vitamin C and vitamin E and restores their antioxidant capabilities; and

- ameliorates the adverse effects of chemotherapy.

GSH, AGEs, and Aging

Important studies have shown that GSH can actually reverse the early effects of glycation on myosin (protein in muscle) function. GSH levels in our cells typically decrease as we age, resulting in a gradual decline in immune function. Studies have demonstrated that:

- GSH blood levels decrease 17% between the ages of 40 and 60.

- People with higher levels of GSH have one third the incidence of:

    a. arthritis,

    b. high blood pressure,

    c. heart disease,

    d. circulatory problems,

    e. gastrointestinal distress/stomach problems,

    f. diabetes, and

    g. urinary tract infections.

- GSH added to the white blood cells of elderly people increased immune activity to a level nearly equal to that of much younger people.

- GSH cleanses the GI tract of rancid fat that would otherwise circulate throughout the body, promoting a variety of age-related conditions.

GSH levels also decrease with the onset of age-related conditions. Aging individuals can recover from diseases and accidents like much younger people if they have high GSH levels. Individuals with higher GSH levels in their blood and tissues live longer and healthier lives.

GSH Enhances Immunity

GSH helps regenerate immune cells. Adding GSH to disintegrating cells that have lost their immune activity revives the cells and causes them to become immunoefficient again. Research has also shown that:

- GSH boosts the ability of T-cells to divide, enabling them to mount stronger attacks on foreign invaders;

- GSH is 90% effective in blocking replication of the AIDS virus in test tube experiments; and

- GSH is typically found at low/deficient levels in AIDS patients.

Protecting Your DNA

If you could look at the tips of your chromosomes, you would find strips of DNA called telomeres. Telomeres protect and stabilize DNA and proteins in the cell. These key pieces of DNA are also involved in regulating cell division. In young cells, the enzyme telomerase keeps telomeres from wearing down too much. But as cells divide repeatedly, there is not enough telomerase, so the telomeres grow shorter and the cells age. Each time the cell divides, the telomere shortens, until eventually there is nothing left, making cell division less reliable, and increasing the risk of age-related disorders. Researchers have found that shorter telomeres are associated with shorter lives. In people 60 and older, those with shorter telomeres were three times more likely to die from heart disease and eight times more likely to die from infectious disease.

GSH restores telomerase to normal levels in cells. This is important because telomerase helps build and maintain telomeres in immune cells.

GSH Removes Toxins

GSH helps the body rid itself of:

- organic toxins (e.g., DDT);

- heavy metals like lead, mercury, and cadmium;

- epoxides like glues and resins;

- halides like chloride, iodide, bromide, and fluoride; and

- toxins produced by physical and emotional stress.

GSH strengthens the body in many ways, including this detoxification. It protects and strengthens the body's immune system so that it can withstand assault from these toxins.

When we stress the body, whether from physical or mental stress, we also increase levels of the hormone cortisol, which elevates blood sugar. Chronic stress means chronically elevated cortisol levels, leading to the formation of AGEs and their degenerative effects.

The GSH Breakthrough

Published research has shown that GSH is the most powerful, versatile, and important of the body's self-generated antioxidants. However, plain GSH cannot survive the digestive tract. Even if GSH is injected into the bloodstream (thus bypassing the digestive tract entirely), an enzyme breaks it down quickly. In fact, conventional GSH has only a 1.6-minute half-life when injected into humans.

Three barriers must be overcome if we are going to get undegraded therapeutic levels of GSH into our systems. First, we have to get it past the stomach. Second, once it's in the bloodstream, we must find a way to prevent the enzymes in the blood from breaking it down. Third, we have to make sure it can be absorbed into the cells.

In an unprecedented breakthrough, scientists have now found a way to deliver a superior form of GSH at therapeutic doses. This patent-pending proprietary process allows GSH to enter the cells in a completely active, safe, and effective manner.

Safety Profile

This new form of modified GSH has an exceptional safety profile. Laboratory animals given the human equivalent of 15,000 mg of GSH a day show no ill effects. Humans generally experience GSH many benefits at doses of 300 to 600 mg/day. No toxicity has been found in humans. GSH is so safe, solutions containing it are used to protect the eye during surgery deep inside this most sensitive organ.

See the Resources section for purchasing information.

VITAMIN B_6—ANTIGLYCATING AGENT EXTRAORDINAIRE

The National Institutes of Health (NIH) classifies and describes vitamin B_6 as a water-soluble vitamin existing in three major chemical forms: pyridoxine, pyridoxal, and pyridoxamine. It performs a wide variety of functions in the body, and is essential for good health. For example, vitamin B_6 is needed for more than 100 enzymes involved in protein metabolism. It is also essential for red-blood-cell metabolism; B_6 is necessary for the proper function of the nervous and immune systems; and it is also necessary for the conversion of the amino acid tryptophan to the B vitamin niacin.

In red-blood-cell metabolism, the body needs vitamin B_6 to make hemoglobin, which is found within red blood cells and carries oxygen to tissues. Vitamin B_6 also helps increase the amount of oxygen carried by hemoglobin. A vitamin B_6 deficiency can result in a form of anemia that is similar to iron-deficiency anemia.

In the immune system, vitamin B_6 is important due to its involvement in protein metabolism and cellular growth. As we age, our immune response—a broad term used to describe the biochemical changes that occur in fighting off infections—weakens. Calories, protein, vitamins, and minerals are important to the immune defenses because they promote the growth of white blood cells, which directly fight infections. B_6

helps maintain the health of the lymphoid organs (the thymus, spleen, and lymph nodes), which make the white blood cells. Animal studies show that a vitamin B_6 deficiency can decrease antibody production and suppress the immune response.

Vitamin B_6 also helps maintain normal blood glucose levels. When your calorie intake is low, your body needs vitamin B_6 to help convert stored carbohydrates or other nutrients to glucose to maintain normal blood-glucose levels.

Focusing on Pyridoxamine

Our search to find therapeutic strategies that can reverse the damage caused by AGEs has led us to focus on pyridoxamine, one of the three aforementioned chemical forms of vitamin B_6.

According to research from the experts at International Aging Systems (*www.anti-aging-systems.com*), supplemental pyridoxamine is the rarest form of B_6, possibly because it is significantly more costly than the other forms.

However, important clinical trials have revealed therapeutic properties in pyridoxamine that do not appear to be present in the more commonly available B_6 vitamins.

One of the most noticeable features of pyridoxamine is the fact that it is the **most potent natural substance for inhibiting AGE formation.**

AGE formation occurs in stages, both early and late. Before studies with pyridoxamine, there was no significant therapeutic strategy for late-stage glycation. This is where pyridoxamine has been shown to be most effective. One study, by Booth et al. and published in the *Journal of Biological Chemistry,* stated that ". . . [pyridoxamine] may complement others . . . known to either prevent initial sugar attachment or scavenge highly reactive dicarbonyl intermediates."

In animal models, pyridoxamine has inhibited both the development and the progression of diabetic nephropathy in type 1 and 2 diabetes (nephropathy is a progressive condition in which blood vessels in the kidney become irreparably damaged). Human trials are ongoing but show promise at doses of 50 mg twice daily. Even at 300 mg daily, no serious side effects or contraindications have been observed.

Apart from inhibiting AGE formation, pyridoxamine also "traps" advanced lipoxidation end products (ALEs). This fact has not escaped researchers interested in atherosclerosis, which, as you learned in Chapter Five, is directly linked to AGE formation. In addition, the presence of excess ALEs seems to affect the structure and function of the vascular wall.

Because pyridoxamine helped reduce the formation of ALEs in animal studies, scientists believe that it could help prevent (or slow) the formation of atherosclerosis, which would naturally assist in the avoidance of heart disease.

Further interesting animal experiments with pyridoxamine have shown improvement for kidney disorders, in particular prevention of kidney stones.

To sum it up, pyridoxamine:

- inhibits formation of AGEs;

- is important in both diabetes and atherosclerosis;

- protects against vascular damage;

- may be useful for treating diabetic retinopathy;

- inhibits renal disease and decreases hyperlipidemia in diabetic rats;

- inhibits progression of nephropathy in the diabetic rat;

- inhibits superoxide radicals and prevents lipid peroxidation;

- inhibits chemical modification of proteins;

- restores beta cell function in diabetic studies; and

- inhibits retinopathy and neuropathy in diabetic laboratory studies.

For information on purchasing pyridoxamine, please see the Resources section.

PYCNOGENOL®

While Pycnogenol is commonly known as a superstrength antioxidant, its health benefits reach far beyond its antioxidant capabilities. Published research studies have demonstrated its beneficial effects in cardiovascular and circulatory health, diabetes care, eye health, venous disorders, inflammation, skin care, healthy aging, and menstrual disorders.

A remarkable study published in *Diabetes Care* reported that Pycnogenol delays the uptake of glucose from a meal 190 times more than prescription medications, preventing the typical high-glucose peak in the bloodstream after a meal. This means that it has strong AGE-preventive properties. Although I have reported on Pycnogenol's many health benefits in other books, it was this study that piqued my interest and encouraged me to contact the Hoboken, New Jersey–based North American distributor, Natural Health Science, Inc. (NHS), to learn more.

Pycnogenol has differentiated itself from other ingredients in the marketplace because of its extensive research portfolio. Unfortunately, this is not always the norm when it comes to researching natural substances such as vitamins, antioxidants, botanicals, and so forth. However, NHS is committed to science and research, and works closely with Horphag Research in its research initiatives. Horphag Research, the exclusive worldwide supplier of Pycnogenol, is the driving force behind the science. Over the last 35 years, the company has invested millions of dollars in extensive scientific research to support the ingredient. To date, the research portfolio includes more than 200 scientific publications, including clinical studies and peer-reviewed articles, ensuring Pycnogenol's safety and efficacy. As a proprietary extract, Pycnogenol is a registered trademark, and is protected by several U.S. and international patents. This wealth of solid scientific data has clearly established Pycnogenol as an indispensable therapy in preventing many degenerative diseases associated with aging—including AGEs and all the damage they cause, from diabetes to heart disease.

Barking up the Right Tree

Pycnogenol is a natural plant extract originating from the bark of maritime pine trees, which grow exclusively along the unspoiled coast of southwestern France. The pine trees from which Pycnogenol is produced are grown entirely without pesticides, and no toxic solvents are used during its production. These trees are ideal botanical sources, as the extracted components are not subject to the seasonal variations that most other plants would have been. This enables the supplier to have a high batch-to-batch consistency in its Pycnogenol.

Pycnogenol contains a unique combination of procyanidins, bioflavonoids, and organic acids, which offer extensive natural health benefits. Pycnogenol has four basic properties:

- It's a powerful antioxidant.

- It acts as a natural anti-inflammatory.

- It selectively binds to collagen and elastin.

- It aids in the production of endothelial nitric oxide, which helps vasodilate (expand) blood vessels.

Pycnogenol Increases Insulin Sensitivity

Pycnogenol is also extremely important in AGE prevention because studies show that it helps lower blood glucose (sugar). This offers help for people with prediabetes, metabolic syndrome, and type 2 diabetes. In one study, Pycnogenol was shown to dose-dependently lower blood-sugar levels in 30 type 2 diabetes patients not requiring medication. These patients followed a diet and exercise program during the 9-week trial. Pycnogenol was given in a daily dosage of 50 mg per day for the first 3 weeks. For the next 3 weeks, the dosage was increased to 100 mg, and then to 200 mg for another 3 weeks. A daily dosage of 50 mg Pycnogenol lowered both fasting and postprandial (after a meal) blood glucose significantly compared to baseline levels. The higher dosages of 100- and 200-mg Pycnogenol were even more effective.

This study, published in the medical journal *Diabetes Care*, found that Pycnogenol did not affect insulin levels. Instead it appears to facilitate blood sugar uptake (use) by previously insulin-unresponsive cells. This is a tremendously important tool in our search for safe, natural substances that can help improve insulin sensitivity. It seems miraculous that Pycnogenol can reawaken these dormant cells—in people who have eaten a typical high-sugar American diet for years—and cause them to respond to insulin again.

Pycnogenol may also offer a significant effective nutritional approach for diabetes prevention—a key goal for all of us, adults and children alike. As you have learned in this book, elevated blood glucose fosters AGE formation, resulting in many degenerative diseases and conditions, including diabetes.

Taking the Starch Out

Pycnogenol also significantly delays the absorption of complex sugars such as starch because it potently inhibits the digestive enzyme α-glucosidase in the duodenum (the beginning of the small intestine). This enzyme is necessary for breaking down complex sugars such as those found in starchy carbohydrates, which consist of thousands of glucose molecules.

Because of the large size of the carbohydrates, starchy foods are not bioavailable, and cannot be absorbed into the bloodstream. The enzyme α-glucosidase liberates one glucose molecule after another from the huge carbohydrate molecule. This is a bit like decomposing a building into its individual bricks. Only monomeric (single) sugars, such as glucose and fructose, can enter the bloodstream.

Blocking the Sugar Enzyme

Normal table sugar (sucrose) is a disaccharide consisting of one part glucose and one part fructose. For absorption into the bloodstream, the sucrose must be split into the two individual monomeric molecules. This splitting of the sucrose molecule can be carried out by the enzyme α-glucosidase, or, to a certain extent, by the acid in the stomach. Unlike the absorption of complex carbohydrates, the absorption of sucrose is not dependent upon the activity of α-glucosidase.

When compared to other α-glucosidase inhibitors such as green tea extract, pure catechin, and the oral antidiabetic medication acarbose (Precose®, Glucobay®), Pycnogenol is dramatically *more effective*. Pycnogenol was four times more effective than the green tea extract.

An-All Day Affair

The ability of Pycnogenol to inhibit α-glucosidase is directly related to the size of its procyanidin (one of its ingredients) molecules. When recent pharmacokinetic studies (studies that measure the process by which a drug is absorbed, distributed, metabolized, and eliminated by the body) were conducted on the procyanidin molecules, it was discovered that these molecules remain in the digestive tract a long time before being absorbed into the bloodstream—typically, four to six hours after consumption. Because these large procyanidin molecules remain available in the intestines for a long time, they are able to inhibit the action of the α-glucosidase enzyme. In fact, if Pycnogenol is taken in the morning, it will maintain its enzyme-blocking action and delay sugar absorption through lunchtime.

We know that sugar and starchy carbohydrates make us overweight and lead to metabolic syndrome, diabetes, heart disease, dementia, Alzheimer's disease, memory problems, glycation of organ systems, including the skin, wrinkles, and the entire host of AGE-generated conditions. If we can lower blood sugar and block absorption of starchy carbs before they can be converted into glucose (sugar), we can begin to stop this degenerative cycle.

Pycnogenol—Master Multitasker

The major cardiovascular risk factors in type 2 diabetes that are involved in the development of metabolic syndrome are responsible for the high mortality from cardiovascular disease in diabetes. In addition to lowering blood glucose, Pycnogenol has been shown to affect these risk factors, significantly lowering systolic blood pressure, improving the blood-lipid profile, and normalizing platelet activity in several double-blind, placebo-controlled clinical trials. All this from one supplement seems almost too good to be true—but it is. Pycnogenol offers a multifactorial approach for improving diabetic syndrome and lowering the cardiovascular risk factors in diabetes—a very big deal because the diabetic's greatest mortality risk is from heart disease—that is now known to be directly linked to AGE formation. Pycnogenol provides significant health protection in diabetes, as demonstrated in controlled clinical trials, including:

- Lowering blood glucose;

- Cardiovascular health-risk reduction;

- Improvement of microvascular health problems, including diabetic microangiopathy, foot ulcers, and muscle cramps; and

- Prevention and improvement of diabetic retinopathy.

Skin-Deep Beauty

No discussion of the impressive properties of Pycnogenol would be complete without mentioning its remarkable ability to bind and protect collagen and elastin, key components of skin and connective tissue. Pycnogenol has a high affinity to proteins rich in the amino acid hydroxyproline, which are predominantly the matrix proteins in the skin, collagen and elastin. When Pycnogenol is added to collagen or elastin, a high amount of both collagen and elastin remains tightly bound. In consequence, Pycnogenol also tightly binds to the skin.

Studies have shown that oral supplementation with Pycnogenol, as well as its metabolites, protects collagen and elastin from degradation by enzymes known as matrix metalloproteinases (MMPs). These MMPs influence the balance between collagen degradation and renewal. Pycnogenol's ability to renew skin's collagen can keep skin youthful and supple—the antithesis of stiff, wrinkled skin showing signs of AGE-damaged glycation to the collagen.

The unique combination of Pycnogenol's pharmacological functions provides an unmatched variety of health benefits for skin health. Pycnogenol:

- selectively binds to collagen and elastin, protecting these proteins from degradation, and making skin firmer, while maintaining youthful suppleness and elasticity;

- enhances circulation to the skin, providing a better supply of oxygen and nutrients, and better hydration and waste removal to make skin clear, radiant, and vibrant; and

- is anti-inflammatory so that it prevents redness, dryness, lines, and wrinkles.

Pycnogenol not only protects against collagenase (an enzyme that breaks down collagen), it also increases skin elasticity. In a double-blind, placebo-controlled clinical study with 62 women, a complex formulation with Pycnogenol as the lead active ingredient was shown to increase skin elasticity after six weeks of oral treatment by 9% as compared to the placebo.

Like alpha lipoic acid, Pycnogenol enhances generation of endothelial (cells that line the interior of blood vessels) nitric oxide (NO), which is the key mediator facilitating arterial relaxation, as opposed to the stiffened blood vessels caused by AGEs, which cut down on blood flow. This allows optimal blood flow to be delivered to the skin, ensuring that nutrients come in and wastes go out.

Oral Pycnogenol supplementation was found to increase blood perfusion of the skin, meaning that the skin is receiving optimal blood supply, all-important nutrients, and better hydration to support its vitality. Poor circulation results in a dull, pallid complexion, lacking the healthy radiance of young skin. All organ systems improve with a healthy blood flow. Oxygen partial pressure is increased, and, conversely, carbon dioxide concentration is decreased. This study also demonstrated an improved healing of wounds (ulcers) in individuals with microcirculatory disorders.

Protecting your Assets

We all know the dangers of exposing the skin to UV rays, including the generation of free radicals, which in turn damage skin cells and connective tissues. In advanced stages, these destructive processes can initiate the immune response of sunburn. This activated immune response causes significant damage to the skin, as it creates even more free radicals, as well as the MMPs described on page 163, which further degrade collagen and elastin. Taken together, this immune response harms the skin significantly more than the UV rays alone.

Oral supplementation of healthy volunteers with Pycnogenol has been shown to help prevent UV damage and resulting photoaging. Pycnogenol inhibits the inflammation caused by UV exposure and consequently protects the skin from sunburn.

In preclinical trials Pycnogenol was also demonstrated to be protective against chronic UV exposure–induced skin malignancies. These findings point to significant photoprotective and antiphotoaging effects of Pycnogenol.

Lighten Up

Pycnogenol inhibits melanogenesis (the production of the pigment melanin, responsible for skin color), and lowers skin pigmentation intensity so that skin is more evenly toned. A clinical study has demonstrated that Pycnogenol is effective in lightening overpigmented areas of the skin, brownish spots or patches that women often develop, especially on the face, and much less frequently on other parts of the body. This type of hyperpigmentation of certain skin areas is known in dermatology as chloasma or melasma.

This phenomenon often affects young mothers or women taking contraceptive hormones. It has also been noted that oxidative stress is involved in the overproduction of skin pigments. Exposure to sunlight greatly contributes to oxidative stress. In attempts to remove these overpigmented areas, aggressive chemical peeling agents are sometimes applied to the skin, even though some are known to cause irreversible skin damage.

The good news is that a study demonstrated that oral supplementation of 30 women with Pycnogenol for one month reduced the area of skin affected by hyperpigmentation by 37%. And, more important, the average pigmentation intensity of women taking part in the trial was lowered by about 22%. In this study Pycnogenol was found to be a safe and effective way to achieve fair skin free of dark spots and patches without any side effects.

A Symphony of Antioxidants

Pycnogenol achieves its anti-inflammatory potency through its ability to inhibit the transcription factor NF-κB, which governs the pro-inflammatory machinery in immune cells. Oral supplementation of Pycnogenol has been shown to significantly inhibit the trigger NF-κB by 15%.

Pycnogenol is a powerful antioxidant, and can effectively neutralize a broad range of free radicals. It also protects vitamin E from oxidation, and recycles oxidized (spent) vitamin C to its bioactive form.

Pycnogenol is also an important contributor to the antioxidant network in the body, a concept introduced earlier in this chapter. That is, it works on its own as well as in concert with other antioxidants, strengthening and reinforcing their effects. Following oral consumption of Pycnogenol over a period of three weeks, the blood oxygen radical capacity (ORAC) of 25 volunteers increased by 40%. The ORAC is commonly used to measure the antioxidant activity of a food ingredient. The higher the measurement, the better the ORAC value.

See the Resources section for purchasing information of this important nutrient. Also, be sure to look for Pycnogenol® with its registered symbol. This is the one to trust, the one that has had extensive clinical testing, and the one that I recommend.

RESVERATROL—KEY TO A LONGER LIFE SPAN

The American Heritage Medical Dictionary defines resveratrol (3,5,4′-trihydroxystilbene) as a natural compound found in grapes (especially in red wine), mulberries, peanuts, and other plants that may protect against cancer and cardiovascular disease by acting as an antioxidant, antimutagen, and anti-inflammatory. Resveratrol also has strong antifungal properties, and is produced by plants in response to microbial attack.

Most resveratrol supplements are made from either red wine extract or from a Chinese plant known as hu zhang (Polygonum cuspidate, aka giant knotweed).

Research into antioxidants continues to support their importance in both health and longevity, with resveratrol in particular turning in a spectacular anti-aging performance. Resveratrol is a powerful AGE inhibitor that, as numerous studies demonstrate, can increase both your life span and your health span. Studies show that it is neuroprotective, antiviral, and anticancer. It can also boost mitochondria, the energy-producing portion of the cell (more about this later).

In addition to the aforementioned attributes, resveratrol has the ability to lower blood sugar and insulin—key factors in AGE prevention. Some of the most exciting studies with resveratrol are the most recent—in fact, results have been so encouraging, scientists believe that the potential exists for the creation of potent antidotes to many of the diseases of aging.

Resveratrol Fights AGE-generated Diseases

A team of researchers from Harvard Medical School and the National Institute on Aging found that high doses of resveratrol reduced the rate of diabetes, liver problems, and other weight-related problems in obese mice, while at the same time extending their life span.

Compared with obese mice eating a high-fat diet, obese mice eating a high-fat diet plus resveratrol had 31% fewer deaths and lived several months longer—as long as mice on a standard, healthful mouse-chow diet.

However, it wasn't just the longevity factor that made the researchers take notice—as amazing as that was, they also found that the organs of the resveratrol-fed obese mice looked normal, when they should have shown signs of significant AGE-generated degradation.

Cholesterol levels of resveratrol-fed mice showed no improvement; however, this did not appear to impact their overall health.

The resveratrol-treated obese mice were also about as healthy, agile, and active on exercise equipment as their lean counterparts, their high-calorie diet notwithstanding. According to lead author Dr. David Sinclair of Harvard Medical School, "These fat, old mice can perform as well on this skill test as young, lean mice."

Forever Young

Dr. Sinclair also noted that preliminary findings indicate that resveratrol may extend the lives of slim mice as well. Sinclair is the cofounder of Sirtris Pharmaceuticals Inc., which is testing resveratrol against human diabetes. Remember, those with uncontrolled diabetes age at a more accelerated rate than nondiabetics. It is exciting to realize that, if resveratrol can impact the health and longevity of those with many diseases, it should have an even more rejuvenating effect on healthy individuals. Sirtris is engaged in very cutting-edge research in the sirtuin family of genes, which have been shown to have a significant effect on the life span of yeast and nematodes.

The National Institute on Aging found the results so encouraging that it is considering repeating the experiment in rhesus monkeys, since they are a much closer genetic match to humans. The hope, of course, is that results such as these can be replicated in humans.

Putting the Daily Dose in Human Terms

The obese mice eating a high-fat diet plus resveratrol were consuming very large doses of the antifungal anticancer antioxidant, equal to 24 milligrams per kilogram (2.2 pounds) of body weight. Resveratrol supplements typically contain from 10 to 20 mg per capsule, so a 130-lb person would need to take about 94 standard capsules per day, delivering about 1,410 mg of resveratrol, to equal the dose that produced such remarkable results in the mice.

However, in another part of the study, obese mice were given a much lower dose, equaling five mg per kilogram per day. They benefited in ways similar to the higher-dose group, but to a lesser extent. This lower dose level would translate to 295 mg of resveratrol per day for our hypothetical 130-lb person, or about 20 standard resveratrol capsules per day. In fact, Dr. Sinclair and several of his lab associates have been taking daily resveratrol doses equaling five mg per kilogram, with no apparent ill effects.

Downsizing the Supersized—More Remarkable Study Results

In addition to the Harvard study, a recent French study further confirms the anti-aging benefits of resveratrol. Mice fed a high-calorie diet were

also given high doses of resveratrol. Remarkably, the mice had the me-
tabolisms and muscle tissue of young, strong athletes. Starting at around
age 40, human bodies begin a slow downward slide in metabolic effi-
ciency characterized by burgeoning waistlines and reduced strength and
endurance. In fact, the majority of health complaints in middle age concern the age-related decline in metabolism.

As we have learned, the most important metabolic reactions in cells
occur inside their mitochondria, the tiny organelles that retain the genes
and enzymes needed for metabolic reactions, including the conversion of
food molecules to usable forms of energy. This energy is the very foundation of cellular metabolism. A young cell is characterized by optimal energy production. Slow that production and you begin the aging process.
The goal, therefore, is to rev up your cellular metabolism—the chemical
and physiological processes by which the body builds and maintains itself, and by which it breaks down nutrients to produce energy. Collec-
tively, the age- and lifestyle-related declines associated with increased
rates of diabetes and heart disease are grouped under the term "metabolic
syndrome," with which we are all familiar.

Now, exciting research from France strengthens the use of resveratrol as
an important therapeutic strategy against metabolic syndrome. Like marine omega-3s (see Chapter Three), resveratrol is recognized as an ally in
the struggle to avoid these dangerous risk factors. And, like the omega-3s,
resveratrol may help us stop accumulating body fat as we age.

The French team at the Institute of Genetics and Molecular and Cellular Biology, led by Johan Auwerx, Ph.D., just released a resveratrol study
whose results seem as exciting as, if not even more exciting than, the Harvard study mentioned earlier.

We all know that a high-fat, high-calorie diet is the kiss of death—to our
health and our looks. However, the findings from this French study found
that the addition of resveratrol significantly countered these effects. High
oral doses of resveratrol:

- prevented weight gain and reduced the size of fat cells;

- protected the animals in the study from developing metabolic
  syndrome;

- increased the number of energy-producing mitochondria in muscle cells;

- boosted thermogenesis (burning of body fat);

- increased the animals' aerobic capacity (i.e., increased their endurance);

- maintained their cells' sensitivity to insulin, thus moderating blood sugar levels;

- transformed muscle fibers into the "slow" type seen in trained athletes;

- enhanced muscle strength and reduced muscle fatigue;

- improved the animals' coordination;

- did not activate $PGC_1-\alpha$ (a transcriptional coactivator of nuclear receptors important to the regulation of a number of mitochondrial genes involved in oxidative metabolism) in the animals' heart muscles, which could be harmful; and

- produced no adverse effects on the liver or other organs.

I find the results of these studies extremely encouraging. They reiterate the fact that we may be able to treat many degenerative conditions with natural substances—substances that can work physiologically, that is, with the body as opposed to against it. Resveratrol appears to be one of the most important of these substances.

Eat Half as Much—Live Twice as Long

As you have learned in this book, maintaining a healthy weight is critical to the prevention of insulin resistance and AGE formation. This is particularly important as we get older and experience metabolism problems. One method proven to significantly lower blood glucose levels is calorie restriction (CR). Since the 1930s extensive scientific research has shown that calorie-restricted diets improve health and extend life spans of nearly every species tested, including worms, spiders, rodents, dogs, cows, and monkeys.

Prior to these studies with resveratrol and some fascinating studies with niacin-bound chromium (see page 106), the only proven strategy for life extension has been CR and fasting.

Several researchers have investigated intermittent fasting (IF) as a method of calorie restriction to obtain health and longevity benefits. Their findings have indicated that intermittent fasting prevents the progression of type I diabetic nephropathy in rats, and changes in the expression of Sir2 and p53. Both IF and CR are effective in expanding life span.

You should already be aware that a better (i.e., smaller) diet can work wonders for type 2 diabetes and related issues—including a significant reduction in the formation of AGEs. Most advocates of CR recommend cut-

Unlocking the Mystery of Calorie Restriction (CR)

In Chapter One you learned of a nematode worm (*Caenorhabditis elegans*) study in the UK that enhanced levels of a critical enzyme involved in protecting against glycation. This resulted in decreased glycation extending life by 40%.

Working again with the nematode, in a study published in *Nature* and reported by the BBC, researchers in the U.S. uncovered a gene that is helping scientists come closer to solving the mystery of just how CR boosts longevity.

The study revealed that a gene known as pha-4 had a significant effect in extending life span. Andrew Dillin, an author of the paper and an associate professor at the Salk Institute for Biological Studies, said: "If you reduce food too much, you go toward starvation and live less long. If you overeat you will succumb to obesity and have a short life span. Dietary restriction is really a sweet spot between the two, a 60 to 70% reduction in normal food intake. But for 72 years, we have not known how it works.

"This is the first gene we have found that is absolutely essential to the longevity response to dietary restriction," Dillin explained. "We finally have genetic evidence to unravel the underlying molecular program required for increased longevity in response to calorie restriction."

What is interesting about the study is that humans and other mammals also have genes comparable to the pha-4 gene. These genes play a key role in early development, and in later life they are important in the regulation of glucagon, a hormone that has a major role in maintaining blood-glucose levels. This function is of particular importance during times of severe food restriction or fasting.

"Pha-4 may be the primordial gene to help an animal overcome stressful conditions to live a long time through dietary restriction conditions," explained Dr Dillin.

If these types of studies can translate into benefits for humans, scientists will look to developing drugs that imitate the effects of CR without having to cut calories by 60%.

Since humans do not take kindly to CR or fasting, this would be a great benefit. The good news is that we have substances such as resveratrol, which appears to provide similar benefits.

ting between 20 and 40% of your calories. I recommend that you start by simply cutting out high-calorie foods that are devoid of nutrition while eliminating most saturated fats from your diet.

The benefits produced in the mice in the French study by dietary resveratrol stem from its effects on an enzyme called SIRT1, which belongs to a recently discovered family of enzymes called sirtuins (introduced on page 167). Sirtuins are the universal regulators of aging in virtually all living organisms. Prior studies showed that SIRT1 activates a substance called PGC1-α, resulting in excellent anti-aging benefits. PGC1-α:

- stimulates cells to produce more mitochondria, thereby increasing energy in the cell—remember, a young cell is characterized by energy production;

- increases the antioxidant capacity needed to handle the free radicals generated by the extra mitochondria;

- changes the mix of fibers in muscle so that there are more of the "slow" type seen in endurance athletes; and

■ causes "burning" of body fat by increasing thermogenesis in brown adipose tissue.

Critically, the new findings prove that resveratrol activates SIRT1 in living animals, with very real, highly desirable metabolic effects—effects that mimic CR.

Command Central

Evidence indicates that SIRT1 commands the body's metabolic and hormonal settings to switch from reproduction to survival mode when levels of energy expenditure drop in our cells.

It was initially believed that sirtuins' main role was to pull key molecules off the proteins that surround DNA—part of the process by which cells turn their genes on and off. However, researchers have now learned that sirtuins are part of a feedback system that enhances cell survival during times of stress, especially if that stress comes from a lack of food.

As mentioned, CR (see box, page 171) has been proven to extend life span by 50% or more in a variety of creatures, such as flies, worms, and mice. The key is to eat a nutritious diet that contains about 30% fewer calories than would normally be eaten.

Sirtuin enzymes evolved to help us survive during difficult periods such as low food availability or famine. Both hunger and resveratrol activate sirtuin enzymes. Once activated, sirtuins alter proteins that affect the aging process, helping prevent the major degenerative diseases of aging, such as cancer, diabetes, heart disease, and dementia.

As mentioned, since the 1930s it has been known that animals placed on calorie-restricted (CR) diets enjoyed significant improvements in both health and longevity. Unsurprisingly, it was recently discovered that sirtuins play a central role in the molecular mechanisms that produce the benefits of such extreme CR. In fact, some of the key signs of aging may stem from age-related declines in the activity of sirtuin-class enzymes.

We can safely assume that millions will await the results of the inevitable human trials with eager anticipation.

The promise of resveratrol rests on the answers to three key questions:

1. Is there is a minimum intake level below which dietary resveratrol produces no metabolic benefits?

2. Would smaller doses of resveratrol produce metabolic benefits to correspondingly smaller extents?

3. Can scientists modify resveratrol so that it is effective at much smaller doses?

In the meantime, we can enjoy foods and beverages that are rich in resveratrol, such as red wine, purple grape juice, dark grapes, cocoa, tea, and some berries, including bilberries, blueberries, raspberries, cranberries, and mulberries. Purchase organic fruit so that you can safely eat the skins—in grapes, for example, the resveratrol is concentrated in the skin.

For the best sources of supplemental resveratrol, see the Resources section and follow dosage recommendations on labels.

The goal of increasing people's average health span is a more meaningful one than increasing their average life span. The good news is that the right combination of antioxidants, with resveratrol and omega-3s leading the team, may make it possible to achieve both—a longer and a healthier life.

PART FOUR

Anti-AGE Strategies for the Skin

8

Seven Threats to Youthful Skin

isted in this chapter are seven of the top threats to youthful, beautiful, healthy skin. However, it isn't just skin that suffers from these threats. If AGEs affect skin, be assured that they are also affecting every other organ system in our bodies, from our heart to our eyes, brain, and kidneys. AGEs are totally indiscriminate in their destruction—they are equal-opportunity destroyers, and no part of the mind or body is immune to their destruction. In the next chapter you will learn about the groundbreaking therapies that can now be part of your anti-AGEs regimen to combat these seven threats.

THREAT #1. THE AGE-ACCELERATING DIET

I begin with diet because eating is something we do every day, three or more times a day. Unfortunately, it is often a somewhat mindless action. We blindly reach for a soda (very bad) or a diet soda (equally bad) instead of a bottle of spring water (good). Or we grab a bagel or Danish (equally bad) instead of a bowl of plain yogurt and a piece of fruit (equally good). If you are an American woman anywhere between the ages of 12 and 100, you are probably always trying to lose weight. In this case you might live on rice cakes (AGE accelerators) or green salads (good) but with no-fat dressing (bad—without healthy fats we can't burn fat, and we can't absorb the nutrients and antioxidants in the salad). And so it goes. If we think about our food choices before we make them, becoming aware and mindful of what we are doing, including eating or drinking, our health will improve, our weight will lessen, and our skin will be rejuvenated.

As you will learn, it is not just our waistlines (or lack thereof) that suffer the consequences of poor choices. My research has shown that the best strategy for keeping the body healthy and the skin youthful and radiant is to follow the anti-AGEs diet, which is designed to carefully control blood sugar and insulin levels. Perricone readers will recognize some of these components from the anti-inflammatory diet, but these recommendations have been refined in light of new research into AGEs.

This means that we must avoid the AGE-accelerating, pro-inflammatory foods, which consist of foods that provoke a glycemic response in the body (i.e., cause a rapid rise in blood sugar). These foods include all forms of sugar, processed foods, pasta, breads, pastry, baked goods, and snack foods such as rice and corn cakes, chips, and pretzels. Extensive lists of both the "good" foods and the "bad" foods can be found in Chapter Four. For the most part, I tell my patients that if the food was made by nature and not the laboratory, it is a good, safe, and healthy option (except for the poor potato, which wreaks havoc with our blood glucose). As we have learned in the preceding chapters, darkly browned and charred foods contribute to AGE formation, as do additives such as caramel coloring and all forms of added sugar, including fructose and high-fructose corn syrup.

These "bad" foods cause an inflammatory response, which results in the formation of AGEs and the acceleration of the aging process in all organ systems. This includes our largest and most visible organ, the skin, resulting in inflexibility, wrinkles, sagging, and the loss of firmness, tone, radiance, and texture.

In place of pro-inflammatory foods, we need to choose foods that have anti-inflammatory properties and/or do not promote AGE formation. See the extensive lists of recommended foods in Chapter Four, but for my purposes in this chapter, I provide an overview of the anti-AGEs diet.

First we need adequate protein (lack of protein accelerates aging) so that our cells can repair themselves. Protein is the building block of life, and the proteins in our body can be rapidly degraded by AGEs. Protein cannot be stored in the body, and must be eaten every day at each meal. Fish, shellfish, poultry, eggs, and low-fat dairy products such as yogurt, kefir, and tofu are excellent sources of high-quality protein.

Next we need low-glycemic carbohydrates (those that will not provoke a glycemic response when consumed in moderation). These include brightly colored fresh fruits and vegetables, whole grains such as old-fashioned oatmeal, and legumes such as beans and lentils.

Finally we need to include healthy fats such as the omega-3 essential fatty acids found in wild salmon. Other healthy fats include acai, avocado, extra-virgin olive oil, olives, nuts, and seeds, all of which will help keep the skin supple and wrinkle free.

For beverages, the best choices include pure spring water, tea (including green tea), and an occasional glass of red wine if you drink wine. I am no fan of diet beverages of any sort—even though there is no sugar or other AGE-promoting sweetener in diet beverages, there may be caramel coloring, dangerous preservatives, and chemical sweeteners with a very questionable safety profile. When possible, try to avoid all kinds of chemicals in your diet, from pesticide residue on nonorganic fruits and vegetables to additives and preservatives. We don't know how our bodies process all of these foreign substances in the long term, and with the high rates of disease such as cancer, which significantly increased after World War II and the advent of processed food, it looks like the answer might be "not too well."

Following the anti-inflammatory diet and lifestyle is the key to health, longevity, mental clarity, well-being, and beautiful, youthful skin. It is one of the best strategies to protect against the dangers of AGE formation and resulting damaging inflammation.

THREAT #2. EXCESSIVE EXPOSURE TO THE SUN

Recent studies have provided evidence that AGEs increase our skin cells' sensitivity to ultraviolet (UV)-induced oxidative stress. AGEs are key mediators in slowing or blocking the growth of skin cells. An important study titled "Photosensitized Growth Inhibition of Cultured Human Skin Cells: Mechanism and Suppression of Oxidative Stress From Solar Irradiation of Glycated Proteins" supports the hypothesis that AGE-modified proteins—in other words, proteins that have become glycated—act as endogenous (internal) sensitizers of photo-oxidative (sunlight) cell damage. That is, they cause the skin cells to incur even greater damage from sun-induced free radicals than they would if the cells were not debilitated by AGE formation.

Once the skin has become AGE-damaged, it is at increased risk for photoaging and photocarcinogenesis (skin cancer) when it is subjected to free radicals generated by UV light. A suntan is an enzymatic browning reaction to UV light and the enzyme tyrosinase, which is involved in increased melanin production. It is not a true Malliard browning reaction, which requires a temperature of 230° F or more, but it is extremely dangerous nonetheless. Sunbathing and tanning accelerate skin aging and increase the risk of skin cancer at any age—but they are particularly harmful as we age.

By now, just about everyone knows that chronic overexposure to sunlight plays a role in skin aging and the development of skin cancer. In fact, it is UV radiation that is the main environmental factor that causes human skin aging. Human skin, like all other organs, undergoes chronological aging; however, unlike other organs, our skin is also in direct contact with the environment. Thus environmental damage adds an additional dimension to the aging process.

And don't forget that your eyes age too and need protection from the sun. Sunglasses protect your eyes from UV rays and reduce the risk of cataracts. They also protect the tender skin around your eyes from sun exposure. Sunglasses that block both UVA and UVB rays offer the best protection. The majority of sunglasses sold in the U.S., regardless of cost, meet this standard. Wraparound sunglasses work best because they also block UV rays from the side.

UV rays are an invisible form of radiation that can penetrate and change the structure of skin cells. Protection from excessive sun exposure is important all year round, not just during the summer or at the beach; UV rays can cause skin damage during any season or temperature. Any time the sun's UV rays are able to reach the earth, you need to protect yourself from excessive sun exposure. For many health reasons, we do need some sun exposure—just use moderation and avoid the sun during peak hours (10 a.m. to 4 p.m. during daylight saving time and 9 a.m. to 3 p.m. during standard time), the most hazardous for UV exposure in the continental U.S. UV radiation is greatest during late spring and early summer in North America.

Remember: UV rays reach you on cloudy and hazy days as well as on bright, sunny ones. UV rays will also reflect off surfaces like water, cement, sand, and snow.

Like chronological aging, sun-induced skin aging is a cumulative process. It differs from chronological aging, which is dependent upon the passage of time; instead it is dependent upon the individual's skin pigment and degree of sun exposure. Lightly pigmented people who spend a lot of time outdoors, especially those who live in warm climates, will experience the greatest degree of photoaging, which can result in the following:

- AGE formation;

- inhibition of new skin cell growth in skin with AGE formation;

- loss of skin elasticity;

- thinner, more translucent-looking skin;

- wrinkles;

- dry, rough, leathery skin;

- broken capillaries on the face;

- freckles;

- liver spots on the face, backs of hands, arms, chest, and upper back;

- spots or blemishes on the lower legs and arms; and

- skin cancer.

Unfortunately, if you visit any beach from Rio to Daytona, from the Hamptons to St. Tropez, you will see people of all ages baking away in the sun—even after all the publicly disseminated information on the danger of tanning. It is even worse when they are smoking and drinking cocktails at the same time, unwittingly and exponentially ramping up the AGE damage thanks to the deadly AGE-generating aldehydes that come from tobacco and alcohol. Remember, I'm not talking about the healthy kind of sun exposure that we need to absorb vitamin D for strong bones. The danger lies in tanning, and both outdoor tanning and indoor tanning booths are implicated. More than 1 million people visit tanning salons on an average day, according to the American Academy of Dermatology (AAD). But many don't know that indoor tanning devices, such as tanning beds and sunlamps, emit UV radiation that's similar to and sometimes more powerful than the sun's UV radiation.

The Centers for Disease Control (CDC) has this to say about skin cancer: Like any other part of our bodies, skin is a place where cancer can develop. Fortunately, most skin cancer can be cured when discovered early and treated promptly. But if you know the facts about skin cancer, you know that it can also be prevented.

According to the American Cancer Society, 600,000 cases of skin cancer occur every year in the U.S., with an estimated 8,200 ending in death.

When exposed to the sun, our skin can go through a series of changes—both short and long term. In the short term, excessive exposure to the sun produces a damaging double whammy. Sun damage to your skin accelerates the glycation process, while skin proteins modified by glycation sensitize your DNA to the damaging effects of the sun's UV rays.

Over time, sun exposure also helps reduce the skin's collagen levels. The sun's UVA rays generate free radicals that oxidize the proteins, lipids, and DNA in the skin, while UVB rays absorbed by DNA promote the cross-linking of adjacent proteins. The end result is an increase in a destructive enzyme known as MMP (see page 163) and a shortage of the molecule that the body uses to make collagen. Limit unprotected sun exposure to 20 or 30 minutes per day, and protect your skin from the sun (with hats, clothes, and UVA/UVB–blocking sunscreen) at other times, especially during the peak-intensity times mentioned on page 181.

Immediate Effects of Sun Exposure

- *Suntan:* A suntan is not a sign of good health. As a defense mechanism, the body produces a pigment called melanin, which turns the skin brown. Suntanning causes skin to age prematurely.

■ *Sunburn:* Sunburns occur when the body receives excessive amounts of radiation (the full effect of the sun is not realized until 14 to 24 hours later). Along with a sunburn, the skin may blister, which indicates a second-degree burn.

Delayed Effects of Sun Exposure

■ *Skin changes:* Skin can change in several ways. The sun can cause skin to age, wrinkle, thicken, dry out, freckle, blemish, and develop a rough texture.

■ *Skin Cancers:* Skin cancers are caused by excessive exposure to the sun's UV rays. It is important to remember that sunburns are not the only condition that lead to the development of skin cancer. Exposure to UV light, heredity, and environment are also important.

There are three basic types of skin cancer, basal cell carcinoma, squamous cell carcinoma, and melanoma. The first two types are very common and easily curable, while the third type, if not detected early, can be very dangerous and even deadly. Every year approximately 32,000 new cases of melanoma develop, causing about 6,700 deaths.

If you think that wrinkle-related photodamage from UV radiation is a far cry from developing skin cancer, think again. It is the first step on a long and dangerous journey. Use sense when out in the sun.

THREAT #3. STRESS

I believe that stress is the most destructive AGE-accelerating force. It affects everyone, which is why I am devoting significant space to help readers understand all the ramifications of letting stress get the better of us. Stress contributes to a great many negative effects, including the instigation of certain hormonal changes in the body, which rapidly alters the function of the cells in the vital organs. Ultimately, these effects are reflected in the appearance of your skin. As you will learn in this chapter, stress has a direct impact on blood glucose levels and AGE formation through its relation to the stress hormone cortisol.

Stress causes the release of the catabolic (the metabolic process in which materials are degraded or broken down) hormone cortisol. Cortisol is typically secreted in response to physical trauma or prolonged stress. Its functions include controlling inflammation, increasing muscular catabolism, suppressing immune response, and maintaining normal vascular circulation and renal (kidney) function. It also controls glycolysis, the metabolic process that breaks down carbohydrates and sugars so that they can be used by the body. If chronically elevated, it will keep blood sugar elevated and thereby promote AGE formation—this is the major AGE-cortisol connection.

When we have large amounts of cortisol circulating in our bloodstreams for extended periods of time, it is extremely toxic. Our brain cells, or neurons, are extremely sensitive to the effects of cortisol. These high circulating levels of cortisol will cause brain cells to die—in fact, high levels of cortisol can actually shrink your brain. Excess cortisol can also destroy your immune system, shrink other vital organs, decrease your muscle mass, and cause thinning of the skin. It will also accelerate wrinkling and skin aging in general, and will cause the blood vessels under skin to appear more prominent.

Understanding Stress

According to highly informative research compiled by the National Institute of Child Health and Human Development (NICHD) division of the National Institutes of Health, the greatest understanding of stress and its effects has resulted from a theory by George Chrousos, M.D., Chief of the Pediatric and Reproductive Endocrinology Branch at the NICHD, and Philip Gold, M.D., of the Clinical Neuroendocrinology Branch at the National Institute of Mental Health (NIMH), which we share here.

A threat to your life or safety triggers a primal physical response from your body, leaving you breathless, with your heart pounding and mind racing. From deep within your brain, a chemical signal speeds stress hormones through the bloodstream, priming your body to be alert and ready to escape danger. Concentration becomes more focused, reaction time becomes faster, and strength and agility increase. When the stressful situation ends, hormonal signals switch off the stress response, and the body returns to normal.

But in our modern society, stress doesn't always let up. Many of us now harbor anxiety and worry about daily events and relationships. Stress hormones continue to wash through our systems in high levels, never leaving our blood and tissues. And so the stress response that once gave ancient people the speed and endurance to escape life-threatening dangers runs constantly in many modern people and never shuts down.

Research now shows that such long-term activation of the stress response can have a hazardous, even lethal effect on the body, increasing the risk of obesity, metabolic syndrome, heart disease, depression, and a variety of other illnesses. Cortisol is directly linked to the proper metabolism of glucose and the release of insulin to maintain healthy blood-sugar levels. Excess cortisol will result in imbalances in blood sugar such as hyperglycemia, which is directly linked to AGE formation.

Much of the current understanding of stress and its effects has resulted from the theory of Drs. Chrousos and Gold. Their theory explains the complex interplay between the nervous system and the stress hormones— the hormonal system known as the hypothalamic-pituitary-adrenal (HPA) axis. Over the past 20 years, Dr. Chrousos and his colleagues have used the theory to understand a variety of stress-related conditions, including depression, Cushing's syndrome, anorexia nervosa, and chronic fatigue syndrome.

The Stress Circuit

The HPA axis is a feedback loop by which signals from the brain trigger the release of hormones needed to respond to stress. Because of its function, the HPA axis is also sometimes called the "stress circuit."

Briefly, in response to a stress, the brain region known as the hypothalamus releases corticotropin-releasing hormone (CRH). In turn, CRH acts on the pituitary gland, just beneath the brain, triggering the release of another hormone, adrenocorticotropin (ACTH) into the bloodstream. Next, ACTH signals the adrenal glands, which sit atop the kidneys, to release a number of hormonal compounds.

These compounds include epinephrine (formerly known as adrenaline), norepinephrine (formerly known as noradrenaline), and cortisol. All three hormones enable the body to respond to a threat. Norepinephrine and epinephrine increase blood pressure and heart rate, divert blood to the muscles, and speed reaction time. Cortisol, also known as glucocorticoid, releases sugar (in the form of glucose) from the body's reserves so that this essential fuel can be used to power the muscles and the brain. However, high levels of cortisol cause excess sugar in the bloodstream, which in turn promotes AGE formation and AGE-generated inflammation.

Normally, cortisol also exerts a feedback effect to shut down the stress response after the threat has passed, acting upon the hypothalamus and causing it to stop producing CRH.

This stress circuit affects systems throughout the body. The hormones of the HPA axis exert their effect on the autonomic nervous system, which controls such vital functions as heart rate, blood pressure, and digestion. The HPA axis also communicates with several regions of the brain, including the limbic system, which controls motivation and mood; the amygdala, which generates fear in response to danger; and the hippocampus, which plays an important part in memory formation. In addition, the HPA axis is also connected with brain regions that control body temperature, suppress appetite, and control pain.

Similarly, the HPA axis interacts with various other glandular systems, among them those producing reproductive hormones, growth hormones, and thyroid hormones. Once activated, the stress response switches off the hormonal systems regulating growth, reproduction, metabolism, and immunity. In the short term, the response is helpful, allowing us to divert biochemical resources to deal with the threat.

Stress, Heredity, and the Environment

According to Dr. Chrousos, the stress response varies from person to person. Presumably, it is partially influenced by heredity. For example, in most people the HPA axis probably functions appropriately enough, allowing the body to respond to a threat, then switching off when the threat has passed. Due to differences in the genes that control the HPA axis, however, some people may fail to have a strong enough response to a threat, while others may overrespond to even minor threats.

Beyond biological differences, the HPA axis can also alter its functioning in response to environmental influences. The HPA axis may be permanently altered as a result of extreme stress at any time during the life cycle—during adulthood, adolescence, early childhood, or even in the womb.

If there are major stresses in early childhood, the HPA feedback loop becomes stronger and stronger with each new stressful experience. This results in an individual who, by adulthood, has an extremely sensitive stress circuit in place. In life-threatening situations—such as life in a war-torn area—this exaggerated response would help an individual survive. In contemporary society, however, it usually causes the individual to overreact hormonally to comparatively minor situations.

The Gastrointestinal Tract and Stress

As many of us know, stress can also result in digestive problems. The stress circuit influences the stomach and intestines in several ways. First, CRH directly hinders the release of stomach acid and the emptying of the stomach. CRH also directly stimulates the colon, speeding up the emptying of its contents. In addition to the effects of CRH alone on the stomach, the entire HPA axis, through the autonomic nervous system, also hinders stomach acid release and emptying, as well as increasing the movement of the colon.

Also, continual high levels of cortisol—as occur in some forms of depression, or during chronic psychological stress—can increase appetite and lead to weight gain. As we know, excess weight leads to obesity and accelerated AGE formation. Rats given high doses of cortisol for long periods had increased appetites and had larger stores of abdominal fat. The rats also ate heavily when they would normally have been inactive. Overeating at night is also common in people who are under stress.

The Immune System and Stress

The HPA axis also interacts with the immune system, making one more vulnerable to colds, flu, fatigue, and infections.

In response to an infection, or an inflammatory disorder like rheumatoid arthritis, cells of the immune system produce three substances that
cause inflammation: interleukin 1 (IL-1), interleukin 6 (IL-6), and
tumor necrosis factor (TNF). These substances, working either singly or
in combination, cause the release of CRH. IL-6 also promotes the release
of ACTH and cortisol. Cortisol and other compounds then suppress the
release of IL-1, IL-6, and TNF, switching off the inflammatory response.

Ideally, stress hormones switch off an immune response that has run
its course. When the HPA axis is continually running at a high level, however, that switching off can have a downside, leading to decreased ability
to release the interleukins and fight infection.

In addition, the high cortisol levels resulting from prolonged stress
could make the body more susceptible to disease by stopping disease-
fighting white blood cells. Although the necessary studies have not yet
been conducted, Dr. Chrousos considers it possible that this same deac-
tivation of white blood cells might also increase the risk for certain types
of cancer.

Conversely, there is evidence that a depressed HPA axis, resulting in
too little corticosteroid, can lead to a hyperactive immune system and increased risk of developing autoimmune diseases like lupus—diseases in
which the immune system attacks the body's own cells. Overactivation of
the antibody-producing B cells may aggravate conditions like lupus,
which result from an antibody attack on the body's own tissues.

Stress-Related Disorders

One of the major disorders characteristic of an overactive HPA axis is
clinical depression. Dr. Chrousos's research has shown that people with
depression often have a blunted ability to adapt to increases in cortisol.
The body turns on the "fight-or-flight" response, but is prevented from
turning it off again. This produces constant anxiety and overreaction to
stimulation, followed by the paradoxical response called "learned help-
lessness," in which victims apparently lose all motivation.

Hallmarks of this form of depression are anxiety, loss of appetite, loss
of sex drive, rapid heartbeat, high blood pressure, and high cholesterol

and triglyceride levels. People with this condition tend to produce higher than normal levels of CRH. The high levels of CRH are probably due to a combination of environmental and hereditary causes.

However, rather than producing higher amounts of ACTH in response to the higher amounts of CRH, depressed people produce smaller amounts of ACTH, presumably because their hippocampuses have become less sensitive to the higher amounts of CRH. In an apparent attempt to switch off excess CRH production, the systems of people with clinical depression also produce high levels of cortisol. However, by-products of cortisol, produced in response to high levels of cortisol, also depress brain cell activity, acting as sedatives, and perhaps contributing to depression.

Other conditions are also associated with high levels of CRH and cortisol, including anorexia nervosa, malnutrition, obsessive-compulsive disorder, anxiety disorder, alcoholism, alcohol and narcotic withdrawal, poorly controlled diabetes, childhood sexual abuse, and hyperthyroidism. Alcoholism, alcohol use, and poorly controlled diabetes are significant factors in accelerated AGE development. In diabetes, we know that excess cortisol secretion is directly connected to the presence and number of AGE-mediated diabetes complications.

The excessive amount of cortisol produced in patients with any of these conditions is responsible for many observed symptoms. Most of these patients share physiological symptoms including sleep disturbances, loss of libido, loss of appetite, and an increased risk for accumulating abdominal fat and for hardening of the arteries (again rooted in AGE formation) and other forms of cardiovascular disease. These patients may also experience suppression of thyroid hormones and the immune system. Because they are at higher risk for these health problems, such patients are likely to have their life spans shortened by 15 to 20 years if they remain untreated.

While many disorders are caused by an overactive stress system, others are caused by an underactive stress system. For example, in Addison's disease, lack of adequate cortisol causes an increase of pigment in the skin, making the patient appear to have a tan. Other symptoms include fatigue, loss of appetite, weight loss, weakness, loss of body hair, nausea, vomiting, and an intense craving for salt. Lack of the hormone CRH also results in extreme tiredness common to people suffering from chronic fatigue syndrome. Lack of CRH is also central to seasonal affective disorder (SAD), in which fatigue and depression plague patients during winter months.

Dr. Chrousos and his team showed that sudden cessation of CRH production may also cause postpartum depression. In response to CRH produced by the placenta, the mother's system stops manufacturing its own CRH. When the baby is born, the mother's sudden loss of CRH may result in sadness or even severe depression for the mother.

Recently, Dr. Chrousos and his coworkers have also uncovered evidence that frequent insomnia is more than just having difficulty falling asleep. The researchers found that, when compared to people who did not have difficulty falling asleep, insomniacs had higher ACTH and cortisol levels, both in the evening and in the first half of the night. Moreover, the insomniacs with the highest cortisol levels tended to have the greatest difficulty falling asleep.

From their ACTH and cortisol levels, it appears that insomniacs have nervous systems that are on overdrive—alert and ready to deal with a threat—when they should be quieting down. Rather than prescribing hypnotic drugs to regulate the sleep system, the researchers suggested that physicians might have more success prescribing antidepressants to help calm overactive stress systems. Behavioral therapy to help insomniacs relax in the evening might also be useful.

After many years of research into the functioning of the HPA axis, Dr. Chrousos concluded that chronic stress should not be taken lightly or accepted as a fact of life.

"Persistent, unremitting stress leads to a variety of serious health problems," Dr. Chrousos said. "Anyone who suffers from chronic stress needs to take steps to alleviate it, either by learning simple techniques to relax and calm down, or with the help of qualified therapists."

Ecotherapy

When it comes to beating stress the tree huggers of the 1960s may have been onto something.

According to Mind, England and Wales' leading mental health charity, a new study by the University of Essex compared the benefits of a 30-minute walk in a country park with a walk in an indoor shopping center on a group of 20 members of local Mind associations.

After the country walk, 71% reported decreased levels of depression and said they felt less tense, while 90% reported increased self-esteem.

This was in contrast to only 45% who experienced a decrease in depression after the shopping center walk, after which 22% said they actually felt more depressed.

Some 50% also felt more tense, and 44% said their self-esteem had dropped after window-shopping at the center.

The university also conducted a second study, asking 108 people with various mental health problems about their experiences with ecotherapy. An impressive 94% said that green activities had benefited their mental health and lifted their depression, while 90% said the combination of nature and exercise had the greatest effect.

Mind describes ecotherapy as "getting outdoors and getting active in a green environment as a way of boosting mental well-being."

I have frequently advised my patients to get out into the fresh air whenever possible—a park, the beach, or even just a leafy, tree-lined street can fill the bill. Breathing fresh air, especially when compared to breathing stale indoor air, has a very beneficial effect, as does the sun's natural full-spectrum light.

"Ecotherapy," or "green therapy," as it is also known, is being recommended either in addition to, or as an alternative to, conventional drug or psychological therapy. But for our purposes here, I think we can safely say that ecotherapy is a safe, effective, and very enjoyable method for reducing the deadly effects of stress. A walk outside provides benefits that a treadmill cannot.

Recommended ecotherapy activities include outdoor walks, gardening, working on a farm, or any other pleasurable activity that unites physical exertion with nature.

THREAT #4. SMOKING CIGARETTES AND/OR EXPOSURE TO SECONDHAND SMOKE

Before I even begin to talk about how smoking affects the skin, stop and consider this:

- Worldwide, tobacco use causes nearly five million deaths per year.

- Current trends show that tobacco use will cause more than 10 million deaths annually by 2020.

- Cigarette smoking is the leading preventable cause of death in the U.S.

- In the U.S., cigarette smoking is responsible for about one in five deaths annually, or about 438,000 deaths per year.

- An estimated 38,000 of these deaths are the result of secondhand smoke exposure.

- On average, smokers die 13 to 14 years earlier than nonsmokers.

- For every person who dies of a smoking-related disease, 20 people suffer with at least one serious illness from smoking.

- Cigarette smoking increases the length of time that people live with a disability by about two years.

- Nearly 21% of U.S. adults (45.1 million people) are currently cigarette smokers.

Now consider this: As mentioned in Chapters six and seven, tobacco smoke is a significant source of exogenous AGEs—and a highly preventable one at that. Physicians know that smoking is a major risk factor not only for lung disease and cancer, but also for heart attack, stroke, and heart failure. Smoking a single cigarette, passive or secondhand smoking, and chronic smoking all lead to stiffer arteries—a known cause of heart disease and one in which AGEs are directly implicated. This in turn increases resistance in the blood vessels and, therefore, increases the work that the heart must do. The good news is that if you stop smoking now, you can actually return your arteries to their presmoking suppleness. Once you stop smoking, your lungs and arteries begin to respond immediately with positive changes. Within as little as 10 years, your arteries will have been restored to the level of stiffness seen in nonsmokers.

As a dermatologist, I can also attest to the fact that smoking leads to deep wrinkles and leathery skin. If you are a smoker, middle age will start in your early 30s as telltale wrinkles around your mouth and eyes begin to appear. But once you stop smoking, the circulation will immediately begin to improve, and as the blood flow returns, your complexion will begin to lose its gray smoker's pallor.

The National Cancer Institute offers programs to help people stop smoking. You can also learn about the benefits that accrue when you stop, which are immediate and substantial, including the following:

- Almost immediately, a person's circulation begins to improve, and the level of carbon monoxide in the blood begins to decline. (Carbon monoxide, a colorless, odorless gas found in cigarette smoke, reduces the blood's ability to carry oxygen.) A person's pulse rate and blood pressure, which may be abnormally high while smoking, begin to return to normal. Within a few days of quitting, a person's sense of taste and smell return, and breathing becomes increasingly easier.

- People who quit smoking live longer than those who continue to smoke. After 10 to 15 years of not smoking, a previous tobacco user's risk of premature death approaches that of a person who has never smoked. About 10 years after quitting, an ex-smoker's risk of dying from lung cancer is 30 to 50% less than the risk for those who continue to smoke. Women who stop smoking before becoming pregnant or who quit in the first three months of pregnancy can reverse the risk of low birth weight for the baby and reduce other pregnancy-associated risks. Quitting also reduces the risk of other smoking-related diseases, including heart disease and chronic lung disease.

- There are also many benefits to smoking cessation for people who are sick or who have already developed cancer. Smoking cessation reduces the risk of developing infections, such as pneumonia, which often causes death in patients with other existing diseases.

■ Quitting smoking reduces the risk of developing cancer—both lung cancer and other types of cancer—and this benefit increases the longer a person remains smoke free. The risk of premature death and the chance of developing cancer due to cigarette smoking depends on the age at which smoking began, the number of years of smoking, the number of cigarettes smoked per day, and the presence or absence of illness at the time of quitting. For people who have already developed cancer, quitting smoking reduces the risk of developing another primary cancer.

■ Smoking cessation benefits men and women at any age. Some older adults may not perceive the benefits of quitting smoking; however, smokers who quit before age 50 have half the risk of dying in the next 16 years, compared with people who continue to smoke. By age 64 if they continue to abstain, their overall chance of dying is similar to that of people the same age who have never smoked.

■ Older adults who quit smoking also have a reduced risk of dying from coronary heart disease and lung cancer. Additional immediate benefits (such as improved circulation, and increased energy and breathing capacity) are other good reasons for older adults to become smoke free.

According to an excellent article posted at www.lifestyle.simplyantiaging.com/smoking-and-skin-aging/ smoking is a worldwide problem with an amazing 1.1 billion smokers—with 50 million of them in the U.S. Studies show that one in two smokers will die prematurely of a smoking-related condition, and most of these smokers are dying in middle age.

Smoking greatly accelerates AGE formation in all organ systems, including the lungs and cardiovascular system. Cigarette smoke is also highly damaging and aging to the skin, where the damage is immediately visible. When we inhale just one puff of a cigarette, more than a trillion free radicals are produced in our lungs, which then activate the white blood cells lining our arteries and trigger an inflammatory response that

Craving a Smoke? Here's What to Do

Nicotine and Your Body and Mind

- As a smoker, you are used to having a certain level of nicotine in your body. You control that level by how much you smoke, how deeply you inhale the smoke, and the kind of tobacco you use. When you quit, cravings develop when the body wants more nicotine.

- When you are exposed to smoking triggers or even when you use a small amount of nicotine, your mood changes. And cravings for tobacco can go up as well as your heart rate and blood pressure. Cravings are *not* "just in your head."

What To Expect

- Cravings usually begin within an hour or two after you stop smoking, peak for several days, and may last several weeks.

- The urge to smoke will come and go. Your cravings will be strongest in the first week after you quit using tobacco. Cravings usually last only a very brief period of time.

- You may also experience cravings that follow each other in rapid succession. As the days pass, the cravings will get further apart. There is some evidence that mild occasional cravings may last for six months.

What To Do

- Remind yourself that cravings will pass.

- As a substitute for smoking, try chewing on carrots, pickles, sunflower seeds, apples, celery, or sugarless gum or hard candy. Keeping your mouth busy may stop the psychological need to smoke.

- Try this exercise: Take a deep breath through your nose and blow it out slowly through your mouth. Repeat 10 times.

- Avoid situations and activities (such as drinking alcohol) that you normally associate with smoking.

- Take 10 mg of B$_6$ twice per day.

- Take 1000 mg of vitamin C in conjunction with the B$_6$ twice per day. These supplements help quell the craving.

Related Notes

- Nicotine cravings may be reduced by using nicotine-replacement products, which deliver small, steady doses of nicotine into the body. Nicotine-replacement patches, gum, lozenges, nasal spray, and inhalable products appear to be equally effective.

How To Get Help

- If you or someone you know wants help with giving up tobacco, please call the National Cancer Institute's Smoking Quitline toll-free at 877-44U-QUIT (877-448-7848). The information specialists on the Quitline can provide suggestions and support to help smokers break the habit.

- The federal government's smokefree.gov website (www.smoke-free.gov) allows you to choose the help that best fits your needs. You can get immediate assistance:

  - View an online step-by-step cessation guide.

  - Find state quitline telephone numbers.

  - Instant message an expert through NCI's *LiveHelp* service.

  - Download, print, or order publications about quitting smoking.

circulates throughout our body, predisposing us to heart disease. In addition, there is a tremendous inflammatory response in all organs of the body—including the skin. Cigarette smoking depletes the skin of oxygen and vital nutrients, including vitamin C, which is critical in keeping skin youthful, moist, and plumped up. Tobacco also acts as a vasoconstrictor, which means that it causes constriction of blood vessels, reducing local blood flow to an area, and temporarily raising blood pressure. When the blood flow to the skin is reduced, it results in a gray, pallid, lifeless, and unhealthy-looking complexion. Smoking also causes dry, leathery-looking skin, premature deep lines, wrinkles, and loss of radiance.

The carbon monoxide in cigarette smoke is a deadly toxin to the entire body. Smoking (and other forms of tobacco use) places us at an increased risk of lung, mouth, and throat cancer.

I applaud the tremendous antismoking awareness campaign that has been waged for the last three decades. Unfortunately, many major motion pictures continue to show people smoking—often incessantly. This has a very negative effect on children and young people. In fact each day, about 1,140 persons younger than 18 become regular smokers, smoking on a daily basis. One look at the aforementioned statistics should deter anyone from taking up smoking. If you already smoke, now is a good time to give it up, because you can positively reverse many of the damaging effects—and the results will quickly be visible in your face and your energy level.

Women and Tobacco

Smoking takes a particularly severe toll on women. In 2001 the special risks of smoking for women were recognized by the U.S. Surgeon General in a report warning women of the dangers of smoking cigarettes. Similar statements were made by European government bodies and other world authorities.

Cigarette smoking kills an estimated 178,000 women in the U.S. annually. The three leading smoking-related causes of death in women in the U.S. are lung cancer (45,000), heart disease (40,000), and chronic lung disease (42,000).

Here are some facts about women and smoking:

- The nicotine in cigarettes is more addictive for women than for men, and women have much more difficulty quitting smoking than men do.

- Women who smoke have twice the additional risk of heart attacks, strokes, and lung cancer than men who smoke.

- Lung cancer kills more than twice as many American women as breast cancer does, which is currently around 70,000 per year.

■ Smoking is linked to early menopause in women.

■ The aging effect of smoking on the skin is worse for women, who are more likely to develop smoker's face than male smokers are.

■ Ninety percent of all lung cancer deaths in women smokers are attributable to smoking. Since 1950, lung cancer deaths among women have increased by more than 600%. By 1987, lung cancer had surpassed breast cancer as the leading cause of cancer-related deaths in women.

■ Women who smoke have an increased risk of other cancers, including cancers of the oral cavity, pharynx, larynx (voice box), esophagus, pancreas, kidney, bladder, and uterine cervix.

■ Women who smoke double their risk of developing coronary heart disease, and increase by more than tenfold their likelihood of dying from chronic obstructive pulmonary disease.

■ Cigarette smoking increases the risk of infertility, preterm delivery, stillbirth, low birth weight, and sudden infant death syndrome (SIDS).

■ Postmenopausal women who smoke have lower bone density than women who never smoked. Women who smoke also have an increased risk for hip fracture over women who never smoked.

"Smoker's Face" and Other Horrors

The effects of smoking on skin aging have been recognized for a long time. A 1965 study first identified what came to be known as "smoker's face"—gray, pale, and wrinkled skin. In recent years much research has focused on this area, and it's now broadly accepted that the skin is damaged by smoking, making smokers look older than nonsmokers of the same chronological ages. Smoking also stains your teeth an unattractive yellowish brown, and can stain your hands and fingernails too.

The Chief Medical Officer of the UK recently highlighted the link between smoking and skin damage, saying that smoking adds between 10 and 20 years to your natural age. So how does smoking speed up skin damage?

It all starts with the free radicals formed in your body by exposure to tobacco smoke. As we know, free radicals are highly unstable and powerful molecules that cause inflammation, resulting in disease and damage to cell DNA. The cells of your body start behaving erratically, producing a range of responses that make your skin age faster. The most serious skin damage is caused by:

- restricted blood flow through the capillaries (tiny veins near the skin's surface), preventing oxygen and nutrients from getting to the skin;

- increased production of an enzyme that breaks down the supply of collagen—which is vital to the skin's elasticity—to the skin's structure. Collagen decreases with age, but smoking cigarettes accelerates this process.

- reduction of the body's store of vitamin A, which provides protection from skin damage;

- decreased ability to absorb vitamin C, a vital antioxidant for skin protection and health;

- smoke in the air, which has an overall drying effect on the skin's surface (dryness is the opposite of youthfulness in skin); and

- continual puckering from drawing on a cigarette and squinting in reaction to the cigarette smoke, creating deeply wrinkled skin around the eyes and mouth—classic signs of smoker's face.

If that is not enough to make you stop smoking, listen to the words of a senior dermatologist, Professor Antony Young of Guys School of Medicine in London, who was the leader of the team that demonstrated in 2001 how collagen loss was accelerated by smoking: "Smoking exerts such a noticeable effect on the skin that it's often possible to detect whether or not a person is a smoker simply by looking at his or her face. Smokers have more wrinkles, and their skin tends to have a grayish pallor compared to nonsmokers."

As a fellow dermatologist I heartily agree with Professor Young's statement. Just as you can identify people who eat large amounts of high-glycemic carbohydrates by their "doughy" look and lack of facial contours, smokers are immediately identifiable by their unhealthy pallor, wrinkles, sagging, and a thick, leathery look to their skin.

Not Just the Face

Dr. Thomas Stuttaford, medical columnist for the *Times* of London, reported recently on the terrible damage smoking does to the body's connective tissue. "One side effect of smoking that isn't capitalized on as much as it could be and might provide a powerful deterrent is its influence on connective tissue," said Dr. Stuttaford. "Few people realize that if they smoke, their faces will wrinkle 10 years ahead of time, and they are likely in middle age to end up with a face like a wrinkled walnut that would rival that of a bloodhound.

Dr. Stuttaford—like many physicians—isn't one to mince words, especially as far as the effects of smoking are concerned, which are not just internal but highly visible externally. If you want to put a "face" to the ravages of AGEs, just look at a smoker. Remember this key fact: Smoking produces aldehydes, which form AGEs. It isn't just sugar attaching to protein that is responsible for AGEs. As you have learned in this and earlier chapters, eating sugars and starches, drinking alcohol, smoking tobacco, and eating charred or overly cooked foods are all major causes of AGEs.

Ten Years After

When you look at your skin, remember that some damage won't appear until 10 to 20 years after you began to smoke. So if you haven't been smoking that long and you don't see much damage yet, don't assume that it won't happen.

The important thing for your skin and your looks is to stop inflicting continued damage on yourself. If you quit smoking now, you will stop your skin from aging any faster than it normally would. And with proper anti-aging skin care and nutrition, the beauty and vibrancy of healthy skin can be restored.

Secondhand Smoke

Even if you don't smoke, be aware of the dangers of secondhand smoke— which are considerable.

- Secondhand smoke, also known as environmental tobacco smoke, is a complex mixture of gases and particles that includes smoke from the burning cigarette, cigar, or pipe tip (sidestream smoke) and exhaled mainstream smoke.

- Secondhand smoke contains at least 250 chemicals known to be toxic, including more than 50 that can cause cancer.

- Secondhand smoke exposure causes heart disease and lung cancer in nonsmoking adults.

- Nonsmokers who are exposed to secondhand smoke at home or work increase their heart disease risk by 25 to 30% and their lung cancer risk by 20 to 30%.

- Breathing secondhand smoke has immediate harmful effects on the cardiovascular system that can increase the risk of heart attack. People who already have heart disease are at especially high risk.

- Secondhand smoke exposure causes respiratory symptoms in children, and slows their lung growth.

- Secondhand smoke increases sudden infant death syndrome (SIDS), acute respiratory infections, ear problems, and more frequent and more severe asthma attacks in children.

- There is no risk-free level of secondhand smoke exposure. Even brief exposure can be dangerous.

One final chilling note on the skin-damaging effects of smoking. A study conducted in 2002 showed that facial wrinkling, while not yet visible, can be seen under a microscope in smokers as young as 20 years of age.

CELESTE'S STORY

I first met Celeste in Paris during the launch of the NV Perricone line at Sephora France. Celeste is a top editor for the French edition of a major international fashion and beauty magazine. Although my trip was a whirl-wind through France, Italy, and the UK, I had set aside considerable time to spend with journalists, and was happy to meet with Celeste.

After she had completed her interview, Celeste asked, "Dr. Perricone, would you mind if I asked you a personal question, not related to the mag-azine?" I assured her that I would be happy to answer her question, as long as it wasn't too personal. "No, no," she exclaimed in her charming accented English. "We French women do not like the Botox," she con-fided. "We are proud of the character lines in our face. But after listening to you talk about the exciting breakthroughs in helping rejuvenate the skin without needles and such, I wonder, do you think the skin-derived stem-cell extract would work for me?" Celeste also revealed that she had embarked on a new relationship that she hoped would evolve into a seri-ous, long-term commitment. This added further impetus to wanting to look her best.

Celeste had the beauty, glamour, and style that are so inherent in French women—especially Parisians. However, although only 40, Celeste was looking drawn and tired. She was also very thin; no surprise, given her career path. Most of the women and men in the fashion and beauty business are obsessive about their weight, regardless of whether they are in front of the camera, behind it, or chronicling the lives of both. The caloric restriction we wrote about in Chapter Seven is a fully embraced way of life in the fashion industry. Unfortunately, its life-extending capa-bilities are compromised because of often-poor food choices, lack of healthy fats, and a penchant for cigarette smoking, which is also rampant in the industry.

Like many Europeans, Celeste smoked, and this had given her deep lines on her upper lip. The nicotine in tobacco is a vasoconstrictor, which means that it causes blood vessels to narrow, cutting down on the flow of blood to the skin. This had given Celeste's complexion a sallow color, although cleverly concealed by a flawless application of makeup.

To help restore Celeste to at least a semblance of her former beauty, we had to address two key areas:

1. Her diet. Celeste was deficient in protein. Without protein, her cells could not repair themselves. This ongoing protein deficiency was very apparent in her face.

2. Cigarettes are a major source of exogenous AGEs, accelerating signs of aging in face and body. When we inhale just one puff of cigarette smoke, more than a *trillion* free radicals are produced in our lungs, which then trigger an inflammatory response that circulates throughout our body.

Forty is a pivotal age. The lifestyle choices we make then will determine whether we stay healthy, active, and vital for the next four decades and beyond. If Celeste stayed on her present course, her face and body would begin to deteriorate rapidly with each passing year. However, if she started now, we could repair much of the damage on a cellular level; that is, from the inside out. I also had a powerful arsenal of topical anti-inflammatories and other unique topical products to increase blood flow to the skin and decrease inflammation while encouraging the skin to again begin responding to the same level of active molecular signals found in young skin.

"Celeste," I said, "we can greatly improve your skin, and in fact greatly increase your overall vitality, but if you are serious about this you need to alter your diet and stop smoking cigarettes."

Celeste had copies of several of my books, which contained all she needed to know about the right food choices and the foods she should cut back on or eliminate altogether. I felt that she would be an excellent candidate for the stem-cell treatment—but only if she stopped smoking. I told her that I would gladly get her started on the dietary and topical program if she complied.

"I'll do it," Celeste said, with both alacrity and conviction. Even though addiction to nicotine has been compared to dangerous drug addiction, I believed her. I knew that she would make the effort and more than likely succeed. One does not rise to the top in such a tremendously competitive profession as hers without plenty of drive and determination. She further confirmed my belief in her when she told me that her near-legendary energy and drive had been flagging of late, causing her serious concern in both her personal and professional life. I think it was this, more than the desire to look younger, that was her true concern. However, like many type-A personalities, she was loath to ever admit any weakness or frailty, especially with a host of power-hungry, ruthless, and much-younger "Celeste wannabes" nipping at her heels.

For Celeste, the news was very good. The simple dietary changes, in conjunction with the cessation of smoking, would dramatically impact her skin and her energy level. In addition, she would experience the added benefit of greater mental clarity, which is particularly important in her world of deadlines and staying ahead of the competition.

In addition to getting Celeste on a nutritional supplement program, I had her add a combination of mCar (the new version of carnosine), omega-3 essential fatty acids, ProCoQ-10, hylaronic acid, the new modified version of glutathione, and astaxanthin to her regimen. These supplements would decrease skin wrinkling, especially in conjunction with the topicals I recommended.

Having seen it work its magic in cases far worse than Celeste's, I had great confidence in the ability of the skin-derived stem-cell extract, which you will learn about in Chapter Nine, to rejuvenate her face and neck. I created a simple routine for her to follow. In the morning after showering, I had her apply a neuropeptide-rich serum preparation to her skin. Once dry, she was to apply the cream containing the stem-cell extract along with proprietary penetration enhancers to her entire face, including the eye area, neck, and jawline. Because the skin-derived stem-cell extract is in a very emollient and highly penetrating base, no further moisturizing was necessary.

In the evening after thoroughly yet gently cleansing her face with a nondrying antioxidant cleanser, Celeste was to apply an advanced alpha lipoic acid (ALA) formula to her face and neck, and a special advanced ALA eye formula to work through the night, increasing blood flow to the skin; reducing skin discolorations, dark undereye circles, and puffiness in the face and eye area; increasing radiance; and decreasing fine lines and wrinkles. ALA's anti-inflammatory effects combined with the skin-firming effects of DMAE (dimethyl amino ethanol) would be rendered even more effective thanks to the ability of the stem-cell messengers to increase uptake of the key ingredients of the ALA and DMAE in the skin—thereby greatly enhancing their already powerful results.

In lieu of her morning croissant and café au lait, Celeste was to have two omega-3 eggs, a slice of melon, berries, and a cup of green tea with fresh lemon. Lunch was to consist of a Greek Salmon Salad or an Asian Crunch Salad with Grilled Turkey Tenderloin (see these and many other delicious recipes in Chapter Eleven) a piece of fresh fruit, and a glass of spring water. Recommended dinner entrees include poached salmon or other seafood, fresh vegetables, and fresh fruit for dessert. These foods would not cause Celeste to gain weight, but they *would* increase her energy and mental prowess, and help rejuvenate both her face and body. Giving up the coffee would make her significantly less tense, and lower her levels of the stress hormone cortisol, which is known to both shrink the brain and thin the skin.

Celeste and I parted with a promise to meet again in four months time in New York City during Fashion week.

The September morning of the first day of Fashion week dawned bright and crisp, a refreshing change from summer's oppressive heat and humidity. As I drove into Manhattan, I reviewed my busy schedule. In addition to providing annual survival kits for the models (little cans of salmon, bottles of spring water, and pieces of fresh fruit) to help them stay on top of their grueling schedules, I was scheduled to have lunch with Celeste. I was looking forward to the meeting, and wanted to personally thank her for the great feature she wrote about my work in her magazine.

Bryant Park was awash in tents, reminding me of a battlefield in the Middle Ages. Thinking about the wildly competitive fashionistas, all vying for their share of the limelight, made me realize that the analogy was fitting—it was a battlefield, and like a battlefield, it was not without casualties.

The morning passed in a blur, and at noon I made my way to the elegant Bryant Park Grill, where I was scheduled to meet Celeste for lunch. I checked my watch as I anxiously scanned the assemblage of elegantly dressed diners. Celeste was nowhere in sight. As the waiter led me to my table on the rooftop, I savored the beautiful views of the park in the background. As usual, there were no empty tables thanks to the glorious weather. I was starting to think that I may have mixed up the date or time when the waiter came to a stop at a table occupied by a very beautiful and stylish young woman who appeared to be in her early thirties.

"Dr. Perricone," she said, "how delightful to see you again." While I didn't recognize the face, I did recognize the voice. "Celeste!" I exclaimed. I was at a loss for words. "An improvement, yes?" she asked. After a summer holiday, Celeste's light brown hair had taken on many golden highlights, which, in conjunction with the changes in her face, made her almost unrecognizable. The ALA had removed the puffiness and dark circles in the eye area, and its anti-inflammatory effects had reduced the redness and uneven skin tone. As we discussed the many positive changes that she had experienced since we had last met, she told me that within a week of quitting smoking, changing her diet, and using the topicals and supplements, a healthy glow began returning to her skin. This was not an illusion or wishful thinking on her part. ALA's capacity to regulate the production of nitric oxide, which controls blood flow to the skin, helped transform her complexion from dull, pasty, and pale to luminous and glowing. And by quitting cigarettes, she was no longer constricting her blood vessels, another plus.

Many of the fine lines and wrinkles in Celeste's eye and mouth area were greatly diminished, and I knew I was also seeing the effects of the ProCo-Q10, the essential fatty acids, and the astaxanthin supplementation in conjunction with the remarkable rejuvenation abilities of the skin-derived stem-cell extract.

With Celeste, the overall changes were proof that the whole was greater than the sum of its parts. She truly looked like a different person. Gone was the drawn and somewhat haggard facial appearance. In its place was an effervescent and vibrant person who radiated health and vitality. The switch from her former poor eating habits to foods rich in nutrients and healthy fats had also greatly contributed to the change. Celeste appeared clear thinking and focused, and had lost that somewhat manic persona so often prevalent in high-powered executives.

Celeste was now a perfect example of my conviction that true beauty is radiant health. With the right synergy of nutrition, nutritional supplements, and novel topical treatments, miracles can and do happen—and Celeste was living proof of it.

THREAT #5. ALCOHOL

People generally think that alcohol is bad for the skin just because it dehydrates the body. They incorrectly assume that increasing their water intake will counteract the problem. Unfortunately, alcohol creates inflammation throughout the body, including the skin, resulting in effects that far outlast dehydration. The metabolites of alcohol are molecules known as aldehydes. Aldehydes cause damage to the cell plasma membrane and parts of the cell interior. And just like glucose, aldehydes promote AGE formation.

Alcohol causes small blood vessels in the skin to widen, allowing more blood to flow close to the skin's surface. This produces a flushed skin color and a feeling of warmth, which can lead to broken capillaries on the face. Alcohol-induced dehydration also makes the skin more prone to fine lines and wrinkles.

Dullness, enlarged pores, discoloration, sagging, and lack of resilience are some of the short-term and long-term effects of alcohol on the skin. Because alcohol alters blood flow to the skin, it gives an unhealthy appearance that can last for days. An occasional glass of red wine can confer some health benefits for a number of reasons. But as with everything from eating to exercise, moderation is the key. Too much alcohol is highly destructive, promoting AGEs in all organ systems, with a particularly devastating effect on the brain—both short and long term. The National Institutes of Health (NIH) has compiled extensive research on the negative effects of alcohol. As a dermatologist, I can also state that alcohol is highly destructive to the skin.

Alcohol's Damaging Effects on the Brain

Difficulty walking, blurred vision, slurred speech, slowed reaction times, impaired memory: Clearly, alcohol affects the brain. Some of these impairments are detectable after only one or two drinks and quickly resolve when drinking stops. On the other hand, a person who drinks heavily over a long period of time may have brain deficits that persist well after he or she achieves sobriety. Exactly how alcohol affects the brain and the likelihood of reversing the impact of heavy drinking on the brain remain hot topics in alcohol research today.

We do know that heavy drinking may have extensive and far-reaching effects on the brain, ranging from simple slips in memory to permanent and debilitating conditions that require lifetime custodial care. And even moderate drinking leads to short-term impairment, as shown by extensive research on the impact of drinking on driving. We also know that alcohol promotes significant AGE formation thanks to the aldehydes it produces. AGEs cause Alzheimer's, dementia, and a whole host of mental problems, so it is not surprising that alcohol induces mental impairment.

A number of factors influence how and to what extent alcohol affects the brain, including:

- the age at which a person first began drinking, and how long he or she has been drinking;

- how much and how often he or she drinks;

- the person's age, level of education, gender, genetic background, and family history of alcoholism;

- whether he or she is at risk as a result of prenatal alcohol exposure; and

- his or her general health status.

Women and Alcohol

Like tobacco, alcohol use takes a particularly heavy toll on women, which is why lower levels of drinking are recommended for women than for men. Women are at greater risk than men for developing alcohol-related problems. Unfortunately, a woman who both smokes and drinks is creating a veritable AGE factory internally. If you were not motivated to quit before, consider this simple fact. The moment you cease smoking and drinking is the moment your skin and internal organs will begin to regain

Detoxifying Alcohol's Effects

In Chapter 3 I introduced Green Magma and other green foods known for their many health benefits. Green foods are also powerful detoxifying agents and can help counter the negative effects of alcohol. Recent research now suggests that the oxidation product of alcohol, acetaldehyde, may be responsible for cancer and other health problems related to alcohol consumption. Acetaldehyde is toxic to tissues, and may produce genetic mutations by damaging DNA.

Normally, alcohol is metabolized to acetate in the liver by several enzymatic steps. Acetate is subsequently metabolized by tissues outside the liver, via the citric acid cycle, to carbon dioxide and water. However, some people lack the gene that is responsible for the production of the enzyme aldehyde dehydrogenase (ALDH), which converts acetaldehyde into acetate. For those lacking ALDH, drinking alcohol may not only be unpleasant, but may also have both short-term and long-term health consequences. Aside from those who lack the gene that produces ALDH, people who are chronic drinkers and people who occasionally overimbibe may also accumulate a level of acetaldehyde sufficient to cause both nausea and tissue damage.

In fact, researcher Mikko Salaspuro, M.D., Ph.D., professor (chair) of Substance Abuse Medicine at the University of Helsinki, noted that acetaldehyde accumulates in the gut when people drink alcohol, and this may have toxic effects on all the tissues of the digestive tract. It is well known that esophageal cancer is linked to heavy alcohol consumption, and acetaldehyde is now thought to be a contributing factor to this disease.

Since acetaldehyde accumulates in the gut during drinking, it may be possible to break down the acetaldehyde by consuming certain drinks or food. The formation of acetaldehyde is prevented by the presence of a unique bioflavonoid called glycosylisovitexin or GIV, found in relatively high concentrations in barley grass juice.

This action of GIV is particularly important in light of research by Finnish researchers showing that acetaldehyde toxicity from alcohol consumption may be a causative factor in cancer of the esophagus and other gastrointestinal tissues. It may also play a role in other cancers. Over the last decade, Professor Takayuki Shibamoto of the Environmental Toxicology Department at the University of California, Davis has published a number of peer-reviewed articles showing that GIV from barley grass juice is very effective at preventing the formation of two types of aldehydes, acetaldehyde and malonaldehyde, which are naturally produced during the oxidation of lipids or alcohol in the body. In 1998, Dr. Shibamoto and colleagues published an article demonstrating the potency of GIV in preventing the formation of acetaldehyde in beer stored at elevated temperatures for more than seven weeks. As little as one microgram of GIV per milliliter of beer inhibited the formation of acetaldehyde by more than 60%, whereas the same amount of the chemical preservative BHT reduced it by only 15%.

Because acetaldehyde is so toxic to the body, it would seem prudent to drink a high-quality barley grass juice such as Green Magma, which contains GIV, before, during, and even after that next alcoholic drink. Green Magma can be taken in supplement form. It is also packaged in individual servings for ease of use.

youthful qualities. If you follow the AGE-prevention advice in this book by increasing intake of the recommended foods and supplements, including the green foods, along with some powerful antiglycating topical treatments, your recovery will be greatly accelerated, and your reward will be highly visible when you look in the mirror.

Alcohol passes through the digestive tract and is dispersed in the water in the body. The more water available, the more diluted the alcohol. As a rule, men weigh more than women, and, pound for pound, women have less water in their bodies than do men. Therefore, a woman's brain and other organs are exposed to more alcohol and to more of the toxic by-products that result when the body breaks down and eliminates alcohol.

Alcoholic women develop cirrhosis (a chronic disease of the liver characterized by the replacement of normal tissue with fibrous tissue and the loss of functional liver cells); alcohol-induced damage of the heart muscle (i.e., cardiomyopathy); and nerve damage (e.g., peripheral neuropathy) after fewer years of heavy drinking than do alcoholic men. Studies comparing men and women's sensitivity to alcohol-induced brain damage, however, have not been as conclusive.

Using imaging with computerized tomography, two studies compared brain shrinkage, a common indicator of brain damage, in alcoholic men and women, and reported that male and female alcoholics both showed significantly greater brain shrinkage than did control subjects. The studies also showed that men and women have similar learning and memory problems as a result of heavy drinking. The difference is that alcoholic women reported that they had been drinking excessively for only about half as long as the alcoholic men in these studies. This indicates that women's brains, like their other organs, are more vulnerable to alcohol-induced damage than are men's.

Yet other studies have not shown such definitive findings. In fact, two reports appearing side by side in the *American Journal of Psychiatry* contradicted each other on the question of gender-related vulnerability to brain shrinkage in alcoholism. Clearly, more research is needed on this topic, especially because alcoholic women have received less research attention than have alcoholic men, despite good evidence that women may be more vulnerable to alcohol's effects on many key organ systems than are men.

Age and Alcohol

Aging seems to reduce the body's ability to process alcohol. Older adults reach higher blood alcohol levels even when drinking the same amount as younger people. This is because with aging the amount of water in the body is reduced, and alcohol becomes more concentrated. But even at the same blood alcohol level, older adults may feel some of the effects of alcohol more strongly than do younger people.

THREAT #6: INSUFFICIENT SLEEP

The interaction and synergy among diet and lifestyle and our health, well-being, and longevity hold the key to how well or how poorly we age. Our diet and lifestyle choices impact all areas of our physical and mental health. Now there is new genetic evidence that physiological outputs of the biological clock, like sleep and appetite, are interconnected at the molecular and behavioral levels. Staying up too late, snacking throughout the day, and skipping meals all upset the genes that control daily rhythms in the brain and throughout the body.

When we deliberately deprive ourselves of much-needed sleep, we are actively disrupting both our glucose metabolism and our neuroendocrine system.

Chronic sleep loss is endemic in modern society. Scientific studies are demonstrating the importance of following a circadian rhythm, that is a 24-hour cycle of waking and rising. Although scientists have long been aware of the interaction between sleeping and eating, it is only recently that we have been able to document the potential impact of chronic sleep curtailment on the risk for diabetes and obesity.

Laboratory studies of healthy young adults subjected to sleep deprivation revealed marked alterations in glucose metabolism, including decreased glucose tolerance and insulin sensitivity. The neuroendocrine system, which regulates appetite, was also adversely affected, leading to cravings for fat- and carbohydrate-rich foods, resulting in subsequent weight gain. This gives new meaning to the term "beauty sleep," as we have long known that our cells repair themselves during sleep, resulting in smoother, more radiant skin. When we are sleep deprived, our skin takes on a pasty, puffy, more wrinkled appearance, and our formerly svelte figures begin to resemble that famous "doughboy" of baking fame.

A growing body of epidemiological evidence supports an association between short sleep duration and the risk for obesity and diabetes—in fact, chronic sleep loss, whether behavioral or sleep disorder–related, may represent a risk factor for weight gain, insulin resistance, and type 2 diabetes. Not getting enough sleep will result in elevated levels of the stress hormone cortisol, lead to inefficient glucose metabolism, encourage weight gain, and accelerate aging and the formation of AGEs.

Sleep Disruption May Increase Risk of Heart Disease

Glycated proteins (AGEs) have also been linked to dangerous blood clots. According to a new study published in the medical journal *Chest*, and reported by Reuter's Health, healthy people who experience sleep disruptions at night appear to have an increased risk for factors associated with the development of a blood clot, also referred to as a thrombus.

"There is an extensive literature demonstrating that sleep disruption is associated with increased coronary artery disease risk, but the possible mechanism for that association has been unclear," lead author Dr. Joel E. Dimsdale, of the University of California San Diego, told Reuters Health.

"In previous work, we have found that sleep disruption was associated with procoagulant activity in patients with obstructive sleep apnea and in patients facing major life stress," he continued. "The current study reports similar findings even in a relatively healthy population."

Dimsdale and colleagues tried to learn whether sleep disruptions, verified by polysomnography, were associated with increased levels of prothrombotic factors previously shown to predict the risk of coronary artery disease. A polysomnograph, conducted in a sleep laboratory, involves the measurement of brain waves to record sleep cycles and stages, plus monitoring muscle activity, eye movement, breathing rate, blood pressure, blood oxygen levels, and heart rate. The patient is also directly observed during sleep.

A total of 135 unmedicated subjects, an average of 37 years old, without a history of sleep disorders, underwent full-night polysomnography. Blood levels of factors associated with blood clotting and oxygen saturation were recorded. The effects of age, gender, ethnicity, body mass index, blood pressure, and smoking history were taken into account.

"Our findings suggest that sleep disruptions, even in a relatively healthy population, are associated with a prothrombotic state that might contribute to coronary artery disease," the authors concluded.

These findings demonstrate that many if not all of the body's organ systems experience negative effects from sleep deprivation or disruptions. Often, getting enough sleep is a conscious choice. We can close that book or shut off the television an hour early and indulge ourselves with a luxurious eight hours of sleep.

Here are six good reasons to follow this advice, courtesy of the Harvard Women's Health Watch:

1. *Learning and memory:* Sleep helps the brain commit new information to memory through a process called memory consolidation. In

studies, people who'd slept after learning a task did better on tests later.

2. *Metabolism and weight:* Chronic sleep deprivation may cause weight gain by affecting the way our bodies process and store carbohydrates, and by altering levels of hormones that affect our appetite.

3. *Safety:* Sleep deficit contributes to a greater tendency to fall asleep during the daytime. These lapses may cause falls and mistakes such as medical errors, air traffic mishaps, and road accidents.

4. *Mood:* Sleep loss may result in irritability, impatience, inability to concentrate, and moodiness. Too little sleep can also leave you too tired to do the things you like to do.

5. *Cardiovascular health:* Serious sleep disorders have been linked to hypertension, increased stress hormone levels, and irregular heartbeat.

6. *Disease:* Sleep deprivation alters immune function, including the activity of the body's killer cells. Keeping up with sleep may also help fight cancer.

Novel Peptide Reduces Stress, Promotes Healthy Sleep

If stress is keeping you awake at night, help may be on the way from a unique food-grade patented product that represents a breakthrough in the field of nutrition.

More than 12 years ago, in partnership with a university in France, a company known as Ingredia discovered a peptide with relaxing properties within a milk protein hydrolysate (a protein hydrolysate is a mixture of amino acids prepared by splitting a protein). Observing the calm state of a baby after drinking milk, researchers attempted to identify a relationship between milk consumption and calmness. Using a well-known digestive enzyme, they developed Lactium®, a functional ingredient that regulates stress symptoms such as weight variations, sleep troubles, cardiovascular disorders, digestive troubles, lack of motivation, irritability, skin troubles, and lack of concentration.

Lactium may be used to help cope with stress from daily life. It can be taken on an as-needed basis to cope with a specific stressful situation, for example, before an exam or important meeting. In these situations, it should be taken at least one hour before the event, and the effect will begin to decrease about six hours after intake.

As a food supplement, the usual recommendation is 167 mg/day. Lactium is effective about one hour after intake. Nevertheless, a real sensation of well-being appears after a few days of treatment. This dosage can be increased if a person is overweight or experiencing a situation that causes an extraordinary level of stress.

The best time to take Lactium is before bedtime. This recommendation is based on the fact that lack of sleep, often provoked by stress from that day, increases one's stress level. Lactium helps people relax and get a better night's sleep, so they'll be better able to meet the demands of the day ahead. Thus, it can help break the vicious cycle of poor sleep and stress.

Clinical studies showed no side effects from Lactium. Lactium regulates the perception of stress, and helps people optimize their abilities and be more reactive. And even at high doses, it has no sedative effect. People who take it feel more relaxed and usually fall asleep more easily at bedtime and/or sleep better.

The major allergenic compounds in milk are proteins, but Lactium is a hydrolysate; hydrolysates are known to be less allergenic than entire proteins. Furthermore, Lactium is lactose free (lactose < 0.5%), so it's OK to take even if you are lactose intolerant.

A good night's sleep will ensure that you awake refreshed, looking radiant and youthful. Adequate sleep is vital to avoid eye area puffiness and maintain vibrant skin. When we look at the hormone parameters during sleep, we find that sleep turns down the negative effects of cortisol and the "bad" neurotransmitters, like epinephrine and norepinephrine, that can be elevated during stress. And growth hormone, which is released during sleep, is the youth hormone. The hormone melatonin is also released, which has a positive effect on the immune system and the skin. It is also during sleep that we rebuild energy reserves and regenerate our body as our cells undergo a process of repair. Studies also show that inadequate sleep leads to unwanted weight gain and a craving for fat-laden and carbohydrate-heavy foods.

Disruptions in the sleep cycle and inadequate sleep cause an increase in the stress hormone cortisol. This, in turn, leads to elevated blood sugar, resulting in AGE formation.

Understanding the Basics of Sleep

Sleep is as essential for your well-being as food and water. Until the 1950s, most people thought of sleep as a passive, dormant part of our daily lives. We now know that our brains are very active during sleep. Moreover, sleep affects our daily functioning and our physical and mental health in many ways that we are just beginning to understand.

Nerve-signaling chemicals called *neurotransmitters* control whether we are asleep or awake by acting on different groups of nerve cells, or neurons, in the brain. Neurons in the brain stem, which connects the brain with the spinal cord, produce neurotransmitters such as serotonin and norepinephrine that keep some parts of the brain active while we are awake. Other neurons at the base of the brain begin signaling when we fall asleep. These neurons appear to "switch off" the signals that keep us awake. Research also suggests that a chemical called adenosine builds up in our blood while we are awake and causes drowsiness. This chemical gradually breaks down while we sleep.

Since sleep and wakefulness are influenced by different neurotransmitter signals in the brain, foods and medicines that change the balance of these signals affect whether we feel alert or drowsy and how well we sleep. Caffeinated drinks such as coffee, and drugs such as diet pills and decongestants, stimulate some parts of the brain and can cause insomnia, or an inability to sleep. Many antidepressants suppress rapid eye movement (REM) sleep. Heavy smokers often sleep very lightly and have reduced amounts of REM sleep. They also tend to wake up after three or four hours of sleep due to nicotine withdrawal. Many people who suffer from insomnia try to solve the problem with alcohol—the so-called nightcap. While alcohol does help people fall into light sleep, it also robs them of REM and the deeper, more restorative stages of sleep. Instead, it keeps them in the lighter stages of sleep, from which they can be awakened easily.

People lose some of the ability to regulate their body temperature during REM, so abnormally hot or cold temperatures in the environment can disrupt this stage of sleep. If our REM sleep is disrupted one night, our bodies don't follow the normal sleep cycle progression the next time we doze off. Instead, we often slip directly into REM sleep and go through extended periods of REM until we "catch up" on this stage of sleep.

People who are under anesthesia or in a coma are often said to be asleep. However, people in these conditions cannot be awakened, and do not produce the complex, active brain wave patterns seen in normal sleep. Instead, their brain waves are very slow and weak, sometimes all but undetectable.

How Much Sleep Do We Need?

The amount of sleep each person needs depends on many factors, including age. Infants generally require about 16 hours a day, while teenagers need about 9 hours on average. For most adults, 7 to 8 hours a night appears to be the best amount of sleep, although some people may need as few as 5 hours or as many as 10 hours of sleep each night. Women in the first three months of pregnancy often need several more hours of sleep than usual. The amount of sleep a person needs also increases if he or she has been deprived of sleep in previous days. Getting too little sleep creates a "sleep debt," which is much like being overdrawn at a bank. Eventually, your body will demand that the debt be repaid. We don't seem to adapt to getting less sleep than we need; while we may get used to a sleep-depriving schedule, our judgment, reaction time, and other functions are still impaired.

People tend to sleep more lightly and for shorter time spans as they get older, although they generally need about the same amount of sleep as they needed in early adulthood. About half of all people over 65 have frequent sleeping problems, such as insomnia, and deep sleep stages in many elderly people often become very short or stop completely. This change may be a normal part of aging, or it may result from medical problems that are common in elderly people and from the medications and other treatments for those problems.

Experts say that if you feel drowsy during the day, even during boring activities, you haven't had enough sleep. If you routinely fall asleep within five minutes of lying down, you probably have severe sleep deprivation, possibly even a sleep disorder. *Microsleeps*, or very brief episodes of sleep in an otherwise awake person, are another mark of sleep deprivation. In many cases, people are not aware that they are experiencing microsleeps. The widespread practice of "burning the candle at both ends" in Western industrialized societies has created so much sleep deprivation that what is really abnormal sleepiness is now almost the norm.

Many studies make it clear that sleep deprivation is dangerous. Sleep-deprived people who are tested using a driving simulator or performing a hand-eye coordination task perform as badly as or worse than those who are intoxicated. Sleep deprivation also magnifies alcohol's effects on the body, so a fatigued person who drinks will become much more impaired than someone who is well rested. Driver fatigue is responsible for an estimated 100,000 motor vehicle accidents and 1500 deaths each year in the U.S., according to the National Highway Traffic Safety Administration. Since drowsiness is the brain's last step before falling asleep, driving while drowsy can—and often does—lead to disaster. Caffeine and other stimulants cannot overcome the effects of severe sleep deprivation. The National Sleep Foundation says that if you have trouble keeping your eyes focused, if you can't stop yawning, or if you can't remember driving the last few miles, you are probably too drowsy to drive safely.

Why We Need Sleep

Although scientists are still trying to learn exactly why people need sleep, animal studies show that sleep is necessary for survival. For example, while rats normally live for two to three years, those deprived of REM sleep survive only about five weeks on average, and rats deprived of all sleep stages live only about three weeks. Sleep-deprived rats also develop abnormally low body temperatures and sores on their tail and paws. The sores may develop because the rats' immune systems become impaired. Some studies suggest that sleep deprivation negatively affects the immune system.

Sleep also appears necessary for our nervous systems to work properly. Too little sleep leaves us drowsy and unable to concentrate the next day. It also leads to impaired memory and physical performance, and reduced ability to carry out math calculations. If sleep deprivation continues, hallucinations and mood swings may develop. Some experts believe sleep gives the neurons that we use while we are awake a chance to shut down and repair themselves. Without sleep, neurons may become so depleted in energy or so polluted with by-products of normal cellular activities that they begin to malfunction. Sleep may also give the brain a chance to exercise important neuronal connections that might otherwise deteriorate from lack of activity.

Deep sleep coincides with the release of growth hormone in children and young adults. Many of the body's cells also show increased production and reduced breakdown of proteins during deep sleep. Since proteins are the building blocks needed for cell growth and for repair of damage from factors like stress and UV rays, deep sleep may truly be "beauty sleep." Activity in parts of the brain that control emotions, decision-making processes, and social interactions is drastically reduced during deep sleep, suggesting that this type of sleep may help people maintain optimal emotional and social functioning while they are awake. A study in rats also showed that certain nerve-signaling patterns that the rats generated during the day were repeated during deep sleep. This pattern repetition may help encode memories and improve learning.

Sleep and Disease

Sleep and sleep-related problems play a role in a large number of human disorders, and affect almost every field of medicine. For example, problems like stroke and asthma attacks tend to occur more frequently during the night and early morning, perhaps due to changes in hormones, heart rate, and other characteristics associated with sleep. Sleep also affects some kinds of epilepsy in complex ways. REM sleep seems to help prevent seizures that begin in one part of the brain from spreading to other brain regions, while deep sleep may promote the spread of these seizures. Sleep deprivation also triggers seizures in people with some types of epilepsy.

Neurons that control sleep interact closely with the immune system. As anyone who has had the flu knows, infectious diseases tend to make us feel sleepy. This probably happens because cytokines, chemicals that our immune systems produce while fighting an infection, are powerful sleep-inducing chemicals. Sleep may help the body conserve energy and other resources that the immune system needs to mount an attack.

THREAT #7. LACK OF EXERCISE

Exercise is vital for your health. Exercise is unsurpassed at lowering our blood sugar—a key strategy in preventing AGE formation. There are mountains of studies proving that exercise can take off pounds, reduce incidence of heart disease, lower blood pressure, improve mood, solve sleep problems, and even cut risks of certain cancers. Exercise will also ensure that you have beautiful skin. Studies have indicated that exercise benefits the skin in much the same way it improves bone and muscle quality. Without regular activity, bones become fragile and muscles atrophy. When the skin of those who exercise regularly is examined under a microscope, the impact of their high fitness levels is clearly apparent. The skin is thicker and has more and healthier collagen, the fibers that give skin its strength and flexibility. Exercise also increases circulation and gives the skin a healthy, radiant glow. As long as we use moderation and don't overdo it, exercise of almost any kind has a powerful, positive, and anti-inflammatory effect on all our cells.

Overexercising will lead to an increase in cortisol levels. As we learned earlier in this chapter, elevated cortisol is highly destructive, leading to elevated blood sugar and AGE formation. Thirty to forty-five minutes per day is all you need.

In Chapter Nine you will learn how to begin to undo the damage caused by the AGE-promoting threats to healthy skin and internal organs.

9

Topical Treatments to Reverse AGEs in the Skin

ost people think that aging skin is caused by chronological age—that is, the older we are in years, the more wrinkled we will be. This is true to a point—a 50-year-old will certainly have more wrinkles than a 20-year-old. However, the truth is not that simple. There are many lifestyle factors that contribute to accelerated aging of skin, such as the seven described in Chapter Eight. These factors significantly accelerate the aging of skin by many mechanisms, including the acceleration of AGE formation, making us look and feel years older than chronological age (and, as we learned in Chapter Two, research done by Dr. Vlassara et al. found high levels of AGEs in healthy young adults—an entirely unexpected and unwelcome phenomenon).

Unfortunately, as we age, AGEs continue to accumulate, and are in part responsible for the loss of the qualities that make skin beautiful. Plastic surgeons and dermatologists alike work hard to restore the look of youth and health—and while we have made great inroads in both disciplines, the overall news is depressing. The damage from accumulated age and accumulated AGEs is highly visible in the skin. No matter how many procedures you have, if there are not some significant changes in diet and lifestyle, it will be difficult to rejuvenate the body. I know, as a physician and a scientist, that true beauty must come from the inside out. As you will learn in this chapter, we have a new, exciting, and incredibly powerful tool that can aid the process. And it is not a wrinkle filler or muscle paralyzer. It goes beyond anything that we have had before. It is the brave new world of stem-cell technology in a new light—safe, nontoxic, noninvasive, and noncontroversial. More about this later in the chapter. But first, let's look at the effects that glycation and AGE formation have on the skin.

If you see a person with deep lines, wrinkles, and grooves in their face; a sallow, leathery look to the skin; and loss of tone and firmness, you are looking at damage from AGEs. There is a strong chance that the internal organs and blood vessels are also damaged. The common denominator for all this damage is, as always, chronic, subclinical inflammation. Remember—when sugar attaches to a protein to create the advanced glycation end products (AGEs), it becomes a factory for the production of inflammatory chemicals.

The good news is that each of the seven of the top threats to healthy, youthful-looking skin outlined in Chapter Eight is in your control—all you have to do is understand how and why each of these seven "deadly sins" takes its toll, and learn the appropriate therapeutic strategy to undo the damage.

HOW AGES DAMAGE SKIN

As we have learned, any one of the seven threats to skin can accelerate aging and AGE formation, not only in the skin, but in the entire body. But for our purposes here we will concentrate on skin.

You learned in Chapter One that glucose, or blood sugar, can exist in two forms. It can either be in a straight line like a string on a table, or it can be in the form of a circle. The greater our sugar and refined starch intake, the more of both types (linear and cyclized glucose) we will have circulating in our blood. At normal body pH (normal physiologic conditions), most of our glucose is in the circular form, which is the more stable formation. However, the remainder of the glucose is in the straight or linear form. This is known as "reactive" glucose. And it is the linear (or bad, if you will) glucose in the blood that reacts with our proteins, resulting in the formation of AGEs.

The Right Antioxidants at the Right Time

In a recent study, scientists put human skin fibroblasts (cells from which collagen and elastin are produced) in a petri dish and exposed them to AGEs. After just 72 hours of exposure to the AGEs, the cells showed damage. It was also discovered that the AGEs dramatically increased free radical damage and inflammation, illustrating just how closely all of these damaging processes are interrelated.

Fortunately, the news was not all bad. When the researchers subsequently exposed the AGE-damaged cells to certain potent antioxidants, including carnosine, much of the cell damage was reversed. This study helps validate the fact that the right antioxidants (which you will learn about in this chapter) given to the skin cells at the right time can help.

In another study, scientists once again placed fibroblasts in a petri dish. They then exposed the cells to a type of AGE known as N-epsilon-(carboxymethyl)lysine or CML-collagen, one of the major products that result from the oxidative modification of glycated proteins (AGEs). Lysine is one of the amino acids that make up collagen; when it is damaged, this lysine molecule alters the collagen, which is then designated CML-collagen. Scientists have identified CML-collagen as a general marker of oxidative stress and long-term damage to proteins in aging, atherosclerosis, and diabetes. When the skin fibroblasts were exposed to CML-collagen, it resulted in apoptosis (death of the skin cells).

As we know, there is strong published data that AGEs accumulate in the dermis, the dense inner layer of skin beneath the epidermis. The dermis is composed of connective tissue, blood and lymph vessels, sweat glands, hair follicles, and an elaborate sensory nerve network. However, that is not the only negative effect on the skin due to the accumulation of AGEs. Scientists have also discovered that there is a receptor (a molecular structure or site on the surface or interior of a cell that binds with substances such as hormones, antigens, drugs, or neurotransmitters) for AGEs that is abundant in skin cells. This receptor is the RAGE, first introduced in Chapter Three, which seriously compounds the problem of AGE-compromised skin. Not only does the skin get cross-linked and bound up by the AGEs, the receptor (RAGE) takes this damaging message to the internal portions of the cells.

AGEs and Collagen

When we were children and had perfect blood pressure and boundless energy, we could play outdoors all day long thanks to a very flexible heart and arteries. This is because our collagen had not yet become "bound up" and stiff.

Collagen is an insoluble protein fiber that is the primary constituent in connective tissue (skin and tendons) and bone. This protein fiber is also found as a support matrix in the arteries. Healthy collagen strands normally slide over one another, which keeps skin elastic. If young people smile or frown, for example, creating lines in the face, the skin will snap back and be smooth again when they stop smiling or frowning. It is the same with our internal organs.

However, as we have gotten older, our collagen has become cross-linked from long-term exposure to the destructive linear sugars. This starts when the collagen becomes attached to one of the bad sugars. It then attaches to another collagen molecule (or other protein) and another and so on in an ever-encroaching matrix.

As more and more AGEs form, accumulating over time, they act like glue or cement, and the result is loss of flexibility in our joints. We also lose flexibility in our arteries, and develop hypertension (high blood pressure). Hypertension can cause a host of dangerous conditions, including blood vessel changes in the back of the eye (retina), abnormal thickening of the heart muscle, kidney failure, and brain damage. When AGEs form in the brain, we suffer from dementia and Alzheimer's disease. When glycation occurs in your skin, the sugar molecules attach themselves to the collagen fibers, where they trigger a series of spontaneous chemical reactions. These reactions culminate in the formation and gradual accumulation of irreversible cross-links between adjoining collagen molecules. This extensive cross-linking of collagen causes the loss of skin elasticity, resulting in wrinkled, sagging skin.

Healthy children, for example, have outstanding learning ability and great memories. They are never stiff or hobbled over, or have difficulty getting up, or feel pain or stiffness in their bodies. Adults, on the other hand, experience all of these symptoms to varying degrees depending on their age and how closely they follow the anti-inflammatory lifestyle that I have been writing about for the past decade. If you feel any of these symptoms, this is a good time to reevaluate food and lifestyle choices before it is too late to undo the damage.

The positive news is that it is possible to reverse these effects. If you follow the advice in this book, you will begin to rapidly see and feel the difference. The longer you follow the advice on how to decrease AGE formation and counter the effects of existing AGEs, the better you will look and feel. Like AGE formation, the results are cumulative—however, in this instance, they get better with time as opposed to worse.

AGEs play a profound part in our eventual decline in health, and this has kept scientists scrambling to find ways to reduce the reactive sugars that are causing the problem. We are also searching for therapeutic strategies that will actually "break" these bonds after they have formed.

TOPICAL SOLUTIONS

Now that we know the seven top threats to aging skin and how AGEs damage skin (see Chapter Eight), it is time to look at solutions to defuse these threats. We know that AGEs take a tremendous toll on our skin. We know this because we can see it every time we look in the mirror. It is their destructive activity that causes our skin to lose its elasticity, suppleness, and tone.

It's important to note that our bodies contain 100 trillion cells that intercommunicate. These cells are in constant communication via "cell" phones that instruct one another what to do, where to do it, and what is going on throughout the body.

The cell phones I am referring to are messenger molecules: peptides, proteins, and lipids (certain fats).

Messenger Molecules in Action

The role of the messenger molecules is to deliver particular messages to receptor sites. The messages delivered depend on the particular neuropeptide, neurotransmitter, or hormone making the call.

When we are young, we have ample messenger molecules. They communicate with the cells in our bodies, including the skin cells, to keep them functioning at optimal levels. However, the level of messenger molecules declines as we age, as do the number of receptor sites. Scientists have long recognized the importance of discovering ways to keep these messenger molecules and receptor sites working properly, because it is the breakdown of this system that is responsible for cellular breakdown in all organ systems.

Armed with this knowledge and the clear understanding of the role of messenger molecules, scientists began to look for ways to keep them functioning at the same youthful and robust levels as those of a young person.

The logical place to look was the stem cells, which secrete the critical messenger molecules necessary for optimal functioning of the body. As a dermatologist, I was naturally drawn to the science of skin stem cells and the possibilities that might exist to restore, repair, and actually *rejuvenate* aging skin. When we consider that the definition of "rejuvenate" is "to make young again; restore to youthful vigor, appearance, etc," we realize that this is a pretty tall order. However, the exciting news is that revolutionary strides are being made in the laboratory.

Freeing the Genie

The goal of the biochemists was to know not only how to repair the skin, but how to actually rejuvenate it. To do so, they took a biotechnological approach to the problem.

The first step was to harvest young adult skin stem cells. The skin samples are taken from behind the ear of healthy young subjects, and the stem cells are then obtained from the skin samples (a process that has no relation to the controversial stem-cell technology that uses embryonic stem cells).

What is so fascinating in this technological breakthrough is that the skin stem cells themselves are used to make the messenger molecules. Once in the laboratory, the youthful skin stem cells are grown in a manner that encourages them to secrete all of the "youthful messengers" necessary to rejuvenate the skin.

The scientists then capture these messengers, purify them, filter them, and process them in such a way that it is only the peptides, proteins, and lipids that are used—*not* the actual skin stem cells themselves. Working closely with these cutting-edge biochemists has enabled me to incorporate this exciting technology into a really revolutionary delivery system for use as a topical treatment for aging skin.

In essence, the "language" of young stem cells has been captured. To me, this is not unlike having captured a genie in a bottle, just waiting to be freed to work its inimitable magic.

Delivering the Messengers

We have skin stem cells in all parts of our skin. Depending on the part of the body being studied, the scientists found that there is a ratio of skin stem cells (SSCs) to regular skin cells of between 1:400 and 1:100,000.

In other words, one lone stem cell is supporting 400 to 100,000 other skin cells. As we get older and our skin cells don't secrete the messengers, and the receptor sites are not functioning as efficiently as they once did, we lose those important messengers that create and maintain healthy, youthful skin—in fact, only 50% or fewer of our skin cells are getting the important messages.

If you are no longer 20, and you are seeing wrinkles, loose skin, and loss of radiance, tone, and texture when you look in the mirror, you are observing the unfortunate end result of your skin cells receiving just half of the rejuvenating SSC messengers that they once did.

In the laboratory, the SSCs are induced to secrete a youthful level of messengers. Those messengers are collected in a sterile environment and then infused into a proprietary formulation designed to deliver the messengers with optimal efficacy. When applied to the face and the body, including the neck, jawline, arms, and legs—in short, anywhere that you choose to revitalize—you will rapidly begin to see results. This skin-derived extract, known as Stimulcell™, is ready, able, and willing to actually replace the lost level of messengers that your older cells are no longer secreting.

Once some of your skin cells begin to make use of these messengers, other skin cells will follow suit. They don't see any difference between the laboratory-produced messengers and the SSC messengers secreted by your body; therefore, they just respond and rejuvenate with all the fervor of the youthful messengers. It's that simple.

In science and mathematics, we use the term "elegant" to describe an experiment, invention, discovery, or concept that combines simplicity, power, and a certain ineffable grace of design. The skin-derived stem-cell extract epitomizes this description. It is simple, elegant, and incredibly efficacious. The implications are not just far-reaching for rejuvenation in skin and internal organ systems, they are also galvanizing and motivating. The possibilities for rejuvenating the mind and body are finally becoming a viable reality thanks to groundbreaking research like this.

The next concern to arise with any substance that is so incredibly active is the safety element. Extensive studies on the messengers' substance, conducted under the most rigorous laboratory procedures, have been conducted. This includes the addition of the skin-derived stem-cell extract to cells in 1,000 times the concentration used in topical preparations. I am happy to report that the results showed the following: Not only was there no damage, no carcinogenic (cancer-causing) properties, and no ill effects whatsoever to the cells tested, it was discovered that the cells that received megadoses of the extract lived longer than untreated cells.

GRACE'S STORY

I first met Grace at our second-year anniversary party for the Perricone flagship store on Madison Avenue. Grace is a very popular and attractive actress, famous for her iconic role as the leading light on a long-running and hugely successful soap opera. She is also renowned for her beautiful skin.

Grace confided that Perricone products were the skin treatments of choice with her fellow actors on the set, and that a number of the cast members were at the party. Although Manhattan is one of the largest and most important cities in the world, in many ways it is also one of the smallest. I was very gratified to see such a show of support and goodwill from so many people in the arts, fashion, beauty, publishing, leisure, travel, media, and entertainment industries in attendance.

As often happens, the conversation turned to the latest breakthroughs in skin rejuvenation and healthy aging technology. Grace explained that she was a huge fan of microdermabrasion and acid peels, believing that they were unsurpassed in helping her reverse the sun damage that she had accrued lying on tropical beaches during hiatus from the show. Although she has since mended her ways, the early damage had been done.

In fact, she told me that she usually had a peel every three to four months, and was going to see her physician that week for the procedure. Glycolic acid peel, or chemical peels, as they are also known, can be any- where from 30% to 70% in strength, depending on what your dermatolo- gist determines is the correct strength. Grace was in the 70% strength level and admitted that, while she loved the ultimate results, the weeks immediately following the peel were difficult, as she experienced a lot of redness, inflammation, and tenderness. This also meant that she had to schedule the peels in the downtimes when she wasn't taping the show to ensure that she had time to recuperate and recover her normal peaches- and-cream complexion.

Because the peels removed the damaged outer layers of the skin, and improved and smoothed skin texture, Grace was willing to endure the af- termath.

My experience working with the skin-derived stem-cell-extract stem- cell messengers encouraged me to suggest to Grace that she try applying the lotion to her skin after the peel to see if it would promote healing. I had seen firsthand the stem cell technology's powerful anti-inflammatory properties as well as its amazing and unique ability to jump-start inactive skin cells to a new level of youthful activity.

I explained to Grace that the topical stem-cell-extract treatment I was referring to did not contain actual stem cells (as explained earlier in the chapter). This is a very important point of differentiation from actual stem-cell therapy, which is a different field altogether.

I instructed Grace to apply the stem-cell-extract lotion after the peel and to use it daily. I asked her to contact me and let me know how she fared.

About a week later, I received a call. "Dr. Perricone," Grace exclaimed, "you will not believe this, but I applied the stem-cell-extract as soon as I returned home from the acid peel procedure. I noticed an almost immediate reduction in my redness and irritation. In fact, even the sensitivity was greatly diminished. Within 24 hours all reactionary symptoms were just about completely gone. I still can't believe it—it usually takes 10 days to two weeks to lose all of the redness and irritation."

Grace went on to add that while she was at her dermatologist's office she had also had a small, strange-looking mole removed from her forearm. Her physician had put a few sutures in after the removal. Once she was back at home Grace also applied the stem-cell-extract lotion to the sutures. Five days later she returned to the office to have the sutures removed. Her dermatologist was extremely surprised to see that there was no closure line from the mole removal—the stem-cell-extract lotion had healed the skin, leaving it as smooth and perfect as skin that had never been sutured. He was also delighted to see that the redness, inflammation, and irritation that Grace usually experienced following a peel had entirely resolved.

Once Grace applied the lotion, the stem-cell messengers began sending their directives to heal the skin just as they would in a young child, rapidly reducing inflammation. The entire healing process was accelerated thanks to the increased number of messengers now reaching receptors in the skin. In addition, collagen and elastin production was accelerated, enhancing the appearance of smooth, firm, supple skin. Anecdotal information shows that Stimulcell™ has great results in treating scars; however, we do not yet have clinical data to support this.

Skin-Derived Stem-Cell Extract's Healing Properties

I have seen and heard many anecdotal stories about the almost miraculous ability of the stem-cell extract to heal postoperative procedures. While these stories are tremendously validating, they are not completely unexpected—although they have exceeded even my high expectations.

The stem-cell extract activates skin cells by rapidly sending out their messengers, just as they would in a healthy young person. As we age, the number and intensity of these messengers declines, causing healing and cellular repair to occur at a much slower and more inefficient rate. In addition, the cellular repair is not as complete or comprehensive as it is in young skin, resulting in many of the signs of aging skin.

Adjunctive therapies such as the stem-cell-extract lotion hold great promise for accelerating healing following surgical procedures, laser treatments, and chemical peels, as well as broad-spectrum application for counteracting the signs of aging in skin. Once the stem-cell extract is applied, it immediately begins to revitalize and reawaken the dormant cells, inciting them to replicate the energy of a young cell. The result? Younger, more beautiful skin, decreased lines and wrinkles, and increased suppleness, tone, firmness, and contour, along with a return to the vibrant radiance of young skin.

I have also found that because the stem-cell extract reenergizes skin cells, intensive antioxidant, anti-inflammatory treatment products such as alpha lipoic acid (ALA), DMAE, vitamin C ester, carnosine, and neuropeptides deliver accelerated benefits to skin. This includes even difficult areas that show early loss of elasticity such as the backs of the hands, elbows, the throat and neck area, the upper lip, and the delicate skin above and below the eye. To learn where to purchase Stimulcell™, see the Resources section.

ALPHA LIPOIC ACID—TOPICAL ANTI-AGES TREATMENT

In addition to the miracle of stem-cell messengers for rejuvenating skin, we also have a number of highly effective topical anti-glycating treatments for skin. Alpha lipoic acid (ALA), a very powerful nutrient when taken as a supplement, is also important as a topical treatment. It is highly recommended as a nutritional supplement (see Chapter Five) because it has powerful antiglycating effects and is an extremely important anti-inflammatory.

ALA increases the cell's ability to take up glucose for metabolism. This removes it from the blood, thereby helping prevent damaging glycation reactions. And because it is both fat and water soluble, it can reach all portions of the cell, providing complete protection. This is true whether it is taken as a supplement or used as a topical. ALA's fat solubility allows it to penetrate into the skin, where it can wield its anti-inflammatory power to great benefit. It protects the cells from free radical damage, and halts the initiation of a skin-damaging inflammatory cascade.

ALA also works synergistically with other antioxidants in the skin, helping decrease the AGE-promoting and pro-inflammatory effects of UV radiation. In addition, ALA can regulate the production of nitric oxide, an important messenger molecule. Nitric acid works in many tissues to regulate a diverse range of physiological processes, including blood flow to the skin. When applied topically, it transforms a dull, sallow, pale complexion to one that is healthy, glowing, and vibrant. It also reduces puffiness in the face and eye area, decreasing fine lines, wrinkles, and pore size.

The ability to be both fat and water soluble is the secret to ALA's ability to rejuvenate the body on a cellular level, because parts of the cell are water soluble and other parts are fat soluble. Since ALA has both properties, it can reach and protect all portions of the cell. In its natural state, ALA is fat soluble. The cell's first line of defense is the outer layer known as the cell plasma membrane, which is actually a lipid (fat) bilayer. This membrane is made up of phospholipids and embedded proteins. The cell plasma membrane is responsible for controlling everything that moves in and out of the cells from nutrients to waste materials. Because it is fat soluble, it is highly susceptible to damage from free radicals. Fortunately, ALA can defend the cell plasma membrane from free radical attack.

Once ALA has entered the cell, it is then changed into a water-soluble nutrient. It can then travel to the watery parts of the cell such as the cytosol, and protect those parts from damage.

The cell also has receptor sites for hormones such as insulin in the cell plasma membrane. Without the right essential fatty acids, these receptor sites will not function properly, preventing glucose from being transported into the cells for energy. These high blood-sugar and insulin levels are pro-inflammatory, and lead to AGE formation. Like essential fatty acids, ALA can also increase insulin sensitivity in the cells. This means that our bodies will metabolize or make our cells more sensitive to insulin, thus allowing our body to metabolize (use up) sugar before it can become attached to collagen and other proteins. Thus ALA is a reliable antiglycating agent—in fact, under certain circumstances it can help reverse AGEs that have already formed.

REJUVENATING SKIN, MUSCLE, AND BONE WITH MICROCURRENTS

As a dermatologist, I not only look for new ways to improve the skin, I also look at the underlying musculature and bone structure. Unfortunately, AGEs take their toll on muscle and bone as well as skin. Fortunately, we have some additional therapeutic strategies that can help undo their damage.

In my last book, *Dr. Perricone's 7 Secrets to Beauty, Health, and Longevity*, I wrote extensively about the importance of both muscle and bone in preserving youthful contours and smooth skin, while maintaining a lifted, firm, and toned face and neck.

To that end, I have been working with a microcurrent machine known as the Ultra, distributed by Ageless Aesthetics and developed by CACI International, a world leader in advanced aesthetic technology.

Understanding Microcurrent

Microcurrent is an electrical current that mimics the electricity found in our bodies. It is only one-millionth of an amp and is subsensory. Clients receiving microcurrent treatments feel little to nothing, with most people experiencing a metallic taste in their mouth as the only indication of the electricity. Microcurrent causes no visible contraction of the muscle because the power is so slight.

Microcurrent:

- increases adenosine triphosphate levels (ATP) by up to 500%. This is a chemical reaction in the body that provides muscle and body energy.

- increases fibroblastic activity by up to 60%. Fibroblast cells are responsible for producing collagen in the skin.

• increases protein synthesis by up to 73%. By increasing protein synthesis, the muscle becomes more "plumped up" and rejuvenated.

• increases membrane transport (cell permeability) by up to 30 to 40%. When the body ages, cells become less permeable, so various functions in the body slow down. Increasing the cell permeability is very successful for treating cellulite. The skin is more moisture retentive and is also rehydrated. In simple terms, this helps cells absorb more nutrients, water, and oxygenated blood, in order to excrete more toxins, prevent fluid retention, and reoxygenate.

• provides dermal nutrition: The Ultra uses a galvanic current to deeply carry specially formulated products into the skin to instantly reduce fine dry lines. This current can also be used with treatments tailored to specific problems such as acne or hyperpigmentation. Using this technique to feed the skin provides improved elasticity and maximum hydration, and helps reduce, or even eliminate, certain visible signs of aging.

• increases collagen and elastin: Exposure to environmental assaults and the natural aging process cause the collagen and elastin that keep our skin resilient to slowly break down. Unfortunately, as we age, the skin's ability to replace these essential materials diminishes, and more gaps and irregularities develop in the collagen mesh, which can lead to wrinkles. Ultra treatments have been shown to amplify the body's own natural production of collagen and elastin to successfully lift away deep lines and shallow wrinkles.

• increases circulation of both blood and lymph flow: Ultra treatments encourage the proper circulation of blood and lymph flow, which are extremely important elements in the condition, color, and overall health of the skin. Once an increase of blood and lymph flow is achieved, the cells receive vital nutrients and oxygen faster, and cell metabolism speeds up, producing healthier and firmer skin.

The Ultra uses a subsensory electric current to reeducate the facial muscles, while improving both the tone and texture of the skin. The process diminishes the appearance of lines and wrinkles, and produces a natural lift without the use of surgery or other invasive methods.

When combined with powerful anti-inflammatory topicals and substances that help reverse the damage from AGEs, the Ultra is a very holistic and natural approach to eliminating many of the signs of aging.

The Ultra can be used on both the face and body, with visible results as early as the first treatment. However, the most dramatic results occur after a complete series of treatments. The number of treatments required depends on the condition of the skin and muscles as well as the desired results. Most people go through an initial series of 6 to 10 treatments and then follow a maintenance schedule of 1 to 2 treatments per month.

These facial treatments are very relaxing and produce little to no sensation. The body treatments are catered to your specific needs and fitness level to ensure that they are both comfortable and effective. At the end of the treatment you can immediately return to your normal activities feeling refreshed and invigorated, with a new, rejuvenated look that goes far deeper than cosmetics.

The Ultra in Action

The Ultra is a combination of three different noninvasive skin-care technologies designed to perform a comprehensive treatment for addressing the premature signs of aging. The Ultra achieves its dramatic results by addressing both the skin tissue and the underlying muscle to both improve the texture of the skin and reeducate the muscles of the face in what has come to be called a "nonsurgical facelift."

First, the Ultra uses microcurrent to address the underlying musculature of the face. As we age, the muscles of our face change in response to the natural aging process, environmental exposure, diet, and lifestyle. Muscles naturally lose ATP, the chemical energy in the muscles that allows them to stay firm. At the same time over- and understimulation of the facial muscles causes deep lines or a slack appearance. Overstimulation comes when we hold the muscles in contraction (e.g., squinting at the computer) and the muscles become shortened, causing a line or wrinkle. Understimulation occurs in the larger muscles of the face, causing them to elongate and create a drooping appearance, as in the cheeks. This is the result of aging muscles producing fewer contractions.

A nonsurgical facelift addresses these issues by manually shortening muscles that have become elongated, and elongating muscles that have become shortened. This is performed through manual manipulation of the muscles with cotton-tipped probes. The elongated muscles are lifted back into position, and the shortened muscles are encouraged to elongate through a stretching massage.

Second, while we are manually manipulating the muscles, we are delivering subsensory microcurrent stimulation that charges the muscle with ATP. This allows the muscles to hold their new positions after the treatment is over. This entire process is called *muscle reeducation*, and it moves the muscles back into their natural youthful position. The treatment is relaxing and, since we are working with the natural lay of the muscles, always produces a result that looks natural—not forced or stretched.

Microcurrent face and body lift technology originated in the spas of Europe, where it became hugely popular, creating great demand for it here in the U.S. This inspired me to install the Ultra at our flagship store on Madison Avenue.

Ultra and Ultrasound

Third, while microcurrent addresses the underlying muscles of the face, the Ultra uses a separate ultrasonic actuator to address problems in the outer layers of the skin. The ultrasonic actuator works with the five characteristics of ultrasound as it relates to improving the skin:

1. *Mechanical action:* The microvibrations of the ultrasound actuator are used to exfoliate dead cells on the upper layer of the skin without the use of acids or abrasive crystals. This type of exfoliation is very beneficial to the skin, and can be used on patients with thin skin and active acne, where microdermabrasion or chemical peels may not be appropriate.

2. *Thermal action:* The molecular friction induced by the ultrasound actuator creates slight warmth in the skin, which dilates the capillaries.

This helps speed up nutrient absorption, lymphatic drainage, and tissue oxygenation.

3. *Metabolic effect:* The ultrasound actuator increases metabolic activity, which is beneficial when the reactivation or acceleration in production of collagen and elastin is the objective (in damaged, aging skins).

4. *Phoretic effect:* The ultrasound actuator increases cell permeability, which, when combined with sonophoresis, allows penetration of targeted topicals into the superficial layers of the skin.

5. *Fibrolytic effect:* Microvibrations produce friction at the dermal level to increase cellular metabolism and renewal. This reduces the formation of fibrous connective tissue often seen in scar tissue and sun-damaged skin.

The Healing Power of Light

The Ultra also uses a combination light therapy/microcurrent handpiece to encourage the reduction of deep lines and wrinkles.

Light has been used for healing for many centuries, starting with the Greeks and Romans, who recognized the positive effects of sunlight. When sunlight strikes the skin, our whole body feels the benefits. Even our brain is affected by sunlight. As scientists have learned more about the nature of light and its positive effects on the body, they have been able to develop techniques and devices that use light as part of the healing process. However, don't take this as a license to worship the sun. We need sun, but we must use it in moderation. Follow the guidelines in Chapter Eight to enjoy the benefits and minimize the risks.

The light used in the Ultra is compressed light of a wavelength from the cold, red part of the spectrum of electromagnetic radiation. It is different from natural light in that it is one precise color; it is coherent (it travels in a straight line), monochromatic (it is a single wavelength) and polarized (it concentrates its beam in a defined location or spot). These properties allow this light to penetrate the surface of the skin with no heating effect, no damage to the skin, and no known side effects. Rather, the Ultra's light directs biostimulative light energy to the body's cells

that the cells then convert into chemical energy to promote natural healing and pain relief.

High-power medical lasers are used to cut through tissue. Light therapy, on the other hand, is used to stimulate tissue repair through a
process of biostimulation.

In the medical setting, light therapy (the application of red and near-
infrared light over injuries or wounds) has been used by physicians to improve soft tissue healing and relieve both acute and chronic pain. Low-level
therapy uses cold (subthermal) light energy to direct biostimulative light
energy to the body's cells without damaging them in any way. In aesthetics,
light therapy has been used to promote the healing of rosacea, sun damage,
and age spots and to stimulate the acupressure points on the face.

How Light Therapy Works

Light therapy supplies energy to the body in the form of nonthermal pho-
tons of light. Light is transmitted through the skin's layers (the dermis,
the epidermis, and the subcutaneous tissue or tissue fat under the skin) at
all wavelengths in the visible spectrum, but light waves in the near-
infrared ranges penetrate the deepest of all of these wavelengths.

When low-level light therapy light waves penetrate deeply into the
skin, they optimize the immune responses of our blood. This has both
anti-inflammatory and immunosuppressive effects. It is a scientific fact
that light transmitted to the blood in this way has positive effects throughout the whole body, supplying vital oxygen and energy to every cell.

Dermatology heads the list of medical disciplines interested in light
therapy, since it is able to stimulate the body's own cell regeneration.
Specialized cells (macrophages) convert the light energy into chemical
energy, therefore increasing the naturally occurring healing mechanisms
of the skin. Light-therapy stimulation results in an increased dilation of
the capillaries, and intercapillary pressure, which leads to an increased
lymphatic flow, stimulation of cellular metabolism, and increased synthesis of proteins. The anti-inflammatory action has been well documented, making light-therapy application particularly beneficial for the
treatment of acne.

Benefits of Light Therapy

- Nonabrasive exfoliation

- Reeducation of facial muscles

- Diminishing of fine lines

- Lifting of heavy jowls and cheeks

- Improvement in definition of jawline

- Softening of deep lines

To learn more about the Ultra, see the Resources section.

THE FUTURE OF BEAUTIFUL SKIN

Thanks to so many emerging technologies, the future looks very positive when it comes to skin rejuvenation. Most important, I do not believe that the future lies in an acceleration of invasive treatments, injectable fillers or neurotoxins, or radical surgery. Great breakthroughs are being made that introduce safe yet genuinely transformative methodologies that not only help restore damaged, aging skin to youthful suppleness, but also reinvigorate the entire body.

As always, we need to remember the holistic nature of the body—every action that we take with diet and lifestyle directly impacts our skin and all our organ systems, for good or ill. We need to be aware of our diet and lifestyle choices. Then and only then can we drastically slow the aging process and its unpleasant consequences.

My goal is not to erase the positive attributes that accrue with age, such as increased wisdom, awareness, tolerance, and spirituality. My goal is to keep you healthy and active for as many decades as possible so that you can continue to contribute to the greater good of the world. We can't accomplish this if we are disempowered by ill health, organ breakdown, loss of mobility, and diminished cognitive abilities.

In Chapter Eleven you will find a great selection of recipes and tips for
turning your kitchen and meal preparation into the ideal haven for generating health, beauty, and longevity for yourself and your loved ones.

One of the most important disease prevention and healing tools we
have is the food we eat.

PART FIVE

The Anti-AGEs Lifestyle

10

Reversing AGE-Related Decline with Exercise

W e all know the importance of exercise. In fact, almost all of us are on some kind of exercise program, usually as a form of weight maintenance. However, there is another very important benefit to be gained from a regular exercise program. Exercise is indispensable when it comes to preventing AGE formation because it enhances glucose uptake, improves insulin sensitivity, and increases lean body mass, which in turn increases overall energy expenditure. Increasing lean body mass and decreasing fat are important because an excess of body fat interferes with the muscles' ability to use insulin, leading to insulin resistance and type 2 diabetes, both of which put you on the fast track for AGE formation.

Because exercise lowers blood sugar, it is an important strategy in slowing AGE formation in people of all ages, including children. In fact, exercise is a tremendously beneficial therapeutic strategy in our quest to prevent and reduce AGE formation.

Most of us desire to be physically fit even if we don't have a clear understanding of what that means. We don't have to be an endurance athlete to be physically fit. We just have to introduce a regular fitness program into our lives and stick with it. The purpose of this chapter is to outline the basics—what you need to know to look and feel your best.

According to the Centers for Disease Control (CDC), physical fitness is defined as "a set of attributes that people have or achieve that relates to the ability to perform physical activity" (USDHHS, 1996). In other words, it is more than being able to run a long distance or lift a lot of weight at the gym. Being fit is not defined only by what kind of activity you do, how long you do it, or at what level of intensity. While these are important measures of fitness, they only address single areas. Overall fitness is made up of five main components:

- *Cardiorespiratory endurance:* Cardiorespiratory endurance (think aerobic) is the ability of the body's circulatory and respiratory systems to supply fuel during sustained physical activity (USDHHS, 1996, as adapted from Corbin & Lindsey, 1994). To improve your cardiorespiratory endurance, do activities that keep your heart rate elevated at a safe level for a sustained length of time (e.g., walking, swimming, or bicycling). The activity you choose does not have to be strenuous to improve your cardiorespiratory endurance. Start slowly with an activity you enjoy, and gradually work up to a more intense pace.

- *Muscular strength:* Muscular strength is the ability of the muscles to exert force during an activity (USDHHS, 1996, as adapted from Wilmore & Costill, 1994). The key to making your muscles stronger is working them against resistance, whether from weights or gravity. If you want to gain muscle strength, try exercises such as lifting weights, strength training (as described in this chapter), or rapidly climbing stairs.

- *Muscular endurance:* Muscular endurance is the ability of the muscles to continue to perform without fatigue during sustained physical activity (USDHHS, 1996, as adapted from Wilmore & Costill, 1994). To improve your muscle endurance, try cardiorespiratory activities such as walking, jogging, bicycling, or dancing.

- *Body composition:* Body composition refers to the relative amount of muscle, fat, bone, and other vital parts of the body (USDHHS, 1996, as adapted from Corbin & Lindsey, 1994). A person's total body weight (what you see on the bathroom scale) may not change over time. But the bathroom scale does not assess how much of that body weight is fat and how much is lean mass (muscle, bone, tendons, and ligaments). Body composition is important to consider for health and managing your weight.

■ *Flexibility:* Flexibility is the range of motion around a joint (USD-HHS, 1996, as adapted from Wilmore & Costill, 1994). Good flexibility in the joints can help prevent injuries through all stages of life. If you want to improve your flexibility, try activities that lengthen the muscles, such as swimming or a basic stretching program. Yoga and Pilates are also great for increasing flexibility.

In order to assess your level of fitness, look at all five components together.

EXERCISING FOR THE HEALTH OF IT

With the huge surge in interest in fitness and exercise, beginning a number of decades ago with the aerobics craze, one would think that fitness had become a way of life in the U.S. Unfortunately, we are less fit as a people than we ever were—even though there is a gym or fitness center on practically every corner. The CDC reports that regular physical activity substantially reduces the risk of dying of coronary heart disease, the nation's leading cause of death, and decreases the risk for stroke, colon cancer, diabetes, and high blood pressure. It also helps control weight; contributes to healthy bones, muscles, and joints; reduces falls among older adults; helps relieve the pain of arthritis; reduces symptoms of anxiety and depression; and is associated with fewer hospitalizations, physician visits, and medications. Exercise lowers blood sugar, a key anti-AGEs and health strategy for diabetics and non-diabetics alike. Remember, whenever you see any type of therapeutic strategy that mentions diabetes, learn all you can and incorporate it into your lifestyle. In this way, you will be learning new and effective methods for decreasing AGEs and mitigating their negative effects.

Physical activity need not be strenuous to be beneficial; people of all ages benefit from participating in regular, moderate-intensity physical activity, such as 30 minutes of brisk walking five or more times a week.

So why aren't we onboard? Despite the proven benefits of physical activity, more than 50% of American adults do not get enough physical activity to provide health benefits. Twenty-five percent of American adults are not active at all in their leisure time. Activity decreases with age, is less common among women than among men, and is less common among those with lower income and less education.

Regular physical activity can improve health and reduce the risk of premature death. In this book our focus is on AGEs. As you will see from this list of benefits, AGE formation is at the very root of each of these diseases. We know that heart disease and stroke are most often caused by atherosclerosis, exacerbated by AGE formation. AGEs also break down muscle, lead to diabetes, obesity, and weight gain, and so on down the list.

Exercise:

- reduces the risk of developing coronary heart disease (CHD) and the risk of dying from CHD;

- reduces the risk of stroke;

- reduces the risk of having a second heart attack in people who have already had one heart attack;

- lowers both total blood cholesterol and triglycerides, and increases high-density lipoproteins (HDL, or "good" cholesterol);

- lowers the risk of developing high blood pressure;

- helps reduce blood pressure in people who already have hypertension (high blood pressure);

- lowers the risk of developing non–insulin dependent (type 2) diabetes;

- reduces the risk of developing colon cancer;

- helps people achieve and maintain a healthy body weight;

- reduces feelings of depression and anxiety;

■ promotes psychological well-being and reduces feelings of stress;

■ helps build and maintain healthy bones, muscles, and joints; and

■ helps older adults become stronger and better able to move about without falling or becoming excessively fatigued.

On the other hand, lack of physical activity can hurt your health. The closer we look at the health risks associated with such a lack, the more convincing it is that Americans who are not yet regularly physically active should become active. Unfortunately, children are now as guilty of inactivity as adults. More than a third of young people in grades 9–12 do not regularly engage in vigorous-intensity physical activity. Daily participation in high school physical education classes dropped from 42% in 1991 to 33.0% in 2005. In 2005, 10% of high school students did not participate in *any* moderate or vigorous physical activity. The U.S. Department of Health and Human Services reports that regular physical activity can help improve the lives of young people beyond its effects on physical health. Although research has not been conducted to conclusively demonstrate a direct link between physical activity and improved academic performance, such a link might be expected.

Participation in physical activity and sports can promote social well-being, as well as good physical and mental health, among people of all ages, including children and teens. Research has shown that students who participate in interscholastic sports are less likely to be regular and heavy smokers or use drugs, and are more likely to stay in school and have good conduct and high academic achievement. As we know, smoking is a great AGE accelerator, as is a diet heavy in the junk food that many children and teens eat in large quantities. An interest in sports and physical activity can get young people started on the road to a long, healthy life and prevent the host of AGE-generated diseases so common today.

Shape Up Your Memory Bank

Exercise also lets us make a very important deposit in our memory banks by reducing the mental disorders, memory loss, and dementia that result from AGEs. We know that AGEs are directly related to all forms of dementia, including the ultimate form: Alzheimer's disease. These mental-health disorders pose a significant public health burden in the U.S., and are a major cause of hospitalization and disability. Mental-health disorders cost approximately $148 billion per year in the U.S. Potentially, increasing physical activity levels in Americans could substantially reduce medical expenditures for mental-health conditions. In the process we could restore our older population to one of bright, active, and mentally engaged people making positive contributions to society well into advanced age. Unfortunately, we now have the opposite, an aging populace ravaged by debilitating mental and physical diseases at an ever-accelerating rate, hastening the breakdown of the health-care system.

The Great Depression

Among people who suffer from mental illness, physical activity appears to improve their ability to perform activities of daily living. Physical activity also has a beneficial effect on adults with affective disorders (a group of disorders characterized by mood disturbances, such as depression or elation). And animal research suggests that exercise may stimulate the growth of new brain cells that enhance memory and learning—two functions hampered by depression. Clinical studies have demonstrated the feasibility and efficacy of exercise as a treatment for depression in older men and women. Currently, National Institute of Mental Health (NIMH) investigators are conducting research comparing the effectiveness of home-based and supervised aerobic exercise to the effectiveness of antidepressants in relieving depression in these groups, and in reducing relapse rates. Other NIMH researchers are studying whether greater exercise levels result in more symptom improvement. While all of this research is commendable, consider what we already know. Chronic high levels of circulating blood sugar and insulin lead to AGE formation. Exercise allows our cells to utilize this blood sugar for energy, making it a surefire way to block AGEs while increasing feelings of physical and mental well-being.

There is no downside to starting a regular exercise program and staying with it for life—and a longer, happier life will be the result.

WALK AWAY THE AGES

The Weight Control Information Network (WIN), a service of the National Institute of Diabetes, Digestive, and Kidney Disorders (NIDDKD), is an outstanding resource of exercise information. Their experts have compiled excellent data on many different forms of exercise, including walking—one of my personal favorite forms of exercise.

While purchasing exercise equipment or joining a gym or health club are viable options, they are not necessary. Walking is one of the finest ways to reduce excess blood sugar—a major culprit in AGEs—and all you need is a comfortable pair of athletic shoes with sturdy heel support and a country trail or city sidewalk. In fact, studies have shown that walking reduces vascular stiffness in healthy middle-aged people. AGEs are directly implicated in atherosclerosis (hardening of the arteries). Keeping our arteries and veins supple so that they carry blood and other fluids to all organ systems is vital to health. The simple act of a daily walk can achieve this, inhibiting the formation of AGEs that harden and stiffen our veins and arteries.

Walking is also one of the easiest ways to be physically active. You can do it almost anywhere and at any time. Walking is also inexpensive. Walking will:

- give you more energy;
- make you feel good;
- help you relax;
- reduce stress;
- help you sleep better;
- tone your muscles;
- help control your appetite; and
- increase the number of calories your body burns.

Another benefit of walking is that we all know how to do it—we don't need to take lessons. In planning your walking program, the experts recommend keeping the following points in mind.

- Leave time in your busy schedule to follow a walking program that will work for you. Choose a safe place to walk. Find a partner or group of people to walk with. Your walking partner(s) should be able to walk with you on the same schedule and at the same speed.

- Wear shoes with thick, flexible soles that will cushion your feet and absorb shock.

- Wear clothes that will keep you dry and comfortable. Look for natural fabrics that allow your skin to breathe.

- For extra warmth in winter, wear a knit cap. To stay cool in summer, wear a baseball cap or visor.

- Do light stretching before and after you walk. Do not bounce when you stretch. Perform slow movements and stretch only as far as you feel comfortable.

- Try to walk every day for a minimum of 30 to 45 minutes. If you can't walk every day, try to walk at least three times per week. Add 2 to 3 minutes per week to the walk. If you walk fewer than three times per week, increase the speed of the walk.

- To avoid stiff or sore muscles or joints, start gradually. Over several weeks, begin walking faster, going farther, and walking for longer periods of time.

- The more you walk, the better you will feel. You also will burn more calories.

GAINING STRENGTH

Ask anyone over 35 or 40 and they will tell you that both their metabolism and their energy have declined significantly since their teens and twenties. It is a fact of life that both will continue to decline with each passing decade. However, there is an antidote to both—exercise, in the form of both aerobics (such as brisk walking) and strength or resistance training.

The real problem that contributes to these declines is the loss of vital muscle mass. In general, Americans lose five pounds of muscle and gain 10 pounds of fat with each decade. Reversing this trend is of the utmost importance if we are to stave off the degenerative conditions associated with aging and AGEs. Aerobic exercise lowers blood glucoses, thereby blocking AGEs and preventing decreased muscle mass. Regular aerobic exercise, such as the walking described above, will increase energy and stamina, and decrease weight gain and the risk of developing heart disease and diabetes.

When it comes to building muscle mass, strength or resistance training has no peer. Both aerobic exercise and strength training improve glucose metabolism and help maintain healthy blood-sugar levels. But strength training has an added benefit: an increase in bone density that helps ward off osteoporosis.

The CDC is an important resource for anyone wishing to start a strength-training program (www.cdc.gov). Not only does it have extensive information on the topic, it also has an interactive program that is easy to follow. It reports that research has shown that strengthening exercises are both safe and effective for women and men of all ages, including those who are not in perfect health. In fact, people with health concerns—including heart disease or arthritis—often benefit the most from an exercise program that includes lifting weights a few times each week. Not only that, nothing firms the body like strength training.

Strength Training Does a Body Good

There are numerous benefits to doing strength training regularly, particularly as we grow older. Not surprisingly, many of them are directly related to reducing the damage caused by AGEs.

- *Arthritis Relief.* Tufts University recently completed a strength-training program with older men and women who had moderate to severe knee osteoarthritis. The results of this 16-week program showed that strength training decreased pain by 43%, increased muscle strength and general physical performance, improved the clinical signs and symptoms of the disease, and decreased disability. The effectiveness of strength training to ease the pain of osteoarthritis was just as potent as, if not more potent than, the effectiveness of medications. Similar effects of strength training have been seen in patients with rheumatoid arthritis, a serious disease in which AGEs can be measured in the synovial fluid (the fluid that lubricates the joint). While strength training cannot reverse the damage to joints caused by arthritis, it *can* strengthen the ligaments, muscles, and tendons around the joints, resulting in less friction and less pain.

■ *Restoration of Balance and Reduction of Falls.* As we age, poor balance and flexibility contribute to falls and broken bones. These fractures can result in significant disability and, in some cases, fatal complications. Strengthening exercises, when done properly and through the full range of motion, increase flexibility and balance, which decrease the likelihood and severity of falls. One study in New Zealand in women 80 years old and older showed a 40% reduction in falls with simple strength and balance training.

■ *Strengthening of Bone.* Postmenopausal women can lose 1 to 2% of their bone mass annually. Results from a study conducted at Tufts University, which were published in the *Journal of the American Medical Association* in 1994, showed that strength training increases bone density and reduces the risk of fractures among women aged 50 to 70.

■ *Proper Weight Maintenance.* Strength training is crucial to weight control, because individuals who have more muscle mass have a higher metabolic rate. Muscle is active tissue that consumes many calories, while stored fat consumes very few calories. Strength training can provide up to a 15% increase in metabolic rate, which is enormously helpful for weight loss and long-term weight control. As we know, AGE promotion is fostered by excess body weight and loss of muscle mass.

■ *Improved Glucose Control.* Studies now show that lifestyle changes such as strength training have a profound impact on helping older diabetic adults manage the disease. People who have metabolic syn-drome or who tend to eat a lot of high-glycemic, AGE-promoting foods will also find significant benefits—including the prevention of diabetes. In a recent study of Hispanic men and women, 16 weeks of strength training produced dramatic improvements in glucose con-trol that were comparable to taking diabetes medication. Addition-ally, the study volunteers were stronger, gained muscle, lost body fat, had less depression, and felt much more self-confident. As we have learned, much of the damage that occurs from diabetes and meta-bolic syndrome is related to AGE formation—if we have less glucose (sugar) circulating, there is less sugar available to attack (and attach to) our body's proteins—and thereby less AGEs and related damage to skin and other organ systems.

■ *Healthy State of Mind.* Strength training provides improvements in depression similar to those provided by antidepressant medications. Currently, it is not known whether this is because people feel better when they are stronger or whether strength training produces a helpful biochemical change in the brain. It is most likely a combina-tion of the two. When older adults participate in strength-training programs, their self-confidence improves, which has a strong im-pact on their overall quality of life.

■ *Sleep Improvement.* People who exercise regularly enjoy improved sleep quality. They fall asleep more quickly, sleep more deeply, awaken less often, and sleep longer. As with depression, the sleep benefits obtained as a result of strength training are comparable to treatment with medication but without the side effects or the ex-pense.

■ *Healthy Heart Tissue.* Strength training is important for cardiac health because heart disease risk is lower when the body is leaner. One study found that cardiac patients gained not only strength and flexibility but also aerobic capacity when they did strength training three times a week as part of their rehabilitation program. This and other studies have prompted the American Heart Association to rec-ommend strength training as a way to reduce the risk of heart disease and as therapy for patients in cardiac rehabilitation programs. Remember that heart disease begins with arterial stiffening related to AGEs. Exercise can help keep the blood vessels (veins and arteries) from stiffening and hardening, helping to avoid heart disease and stroke.

Research and Background of Strength Training

Scientific research has shown that while AGEs accelerate aging, exercise can slow the physiological clock. We know the importance of aerobic exercise (brisk walking, jogging, swimming, etc.) and its many excellent health benefits—it maintains the heart and lungs, and increases cardiovascular fitness and endurance. Studies have shown that lifting weights for 30 minutes two or three times a week increases strength by building muscle mass and bone density.

One 12-month study conducted on postmenopausal women at Tufts University demonstrated 1% gains in hip and spine bone density, 75% increases in strength, and 13% increases in dynamic balance with just two days per week of progressive strength training. The control group had losses in bone density, strength, and balance. Strength-training programs can also have a profound effect on reducing the risk of falls, which translates to fewer fractures.

If you would like to burn more calories; build strong muscles, bones, and joints; improve your physical functioning; and slow AGE formation, strength training is the key. Experts recommend strength training two to three days each week, with one full day of rest between workouts to allow your muscles to recover. If you are new to strength training or physical activity in general, consider hiring a certified personal trainer who can plan an individualized program to help you work out safely and effectively. A personal trainer who has a degree in exercise physiology or who is certified through a national certification program, such as the American College of Sports Medicine or the National Strength and Conditioning Association, may be able to help you reach your physical activity goals.

Helpful tools in our goal to build strong muscles and bones with strengthening exercises include:

- free weights and weight machines;

- resistance bands;

- stability or medicine balls; and

- push-ups and abdominal crunches.

SETTING GOALS TO OVERCOME EXERCISE HURDLES

When taking on any challenge, it's a good idea to define your goals, and the CDC also has excellent advice on defining your exercise goals.

You should identify what you want to accomplish and how you will carry out your plan. This is important when making positive change, and will help you succeed. It is also extremely rewarding, and gives structure to your program. Perhaps most significant is that setting goals gives you something to work toward—it is a terrific motivator. Before starting this program, set short-term and long-term goals. These goals should be *S-M-A-R-T:*

- Specific

- Measurable

- Attainable

- Relevant

- Time based

For example: A *specific* short-term goal may be to start strength training; a long-term goal may be easing the symptoms of arthritis, improving balance, or controlling your weight. This goal is easily *measurable:* Have you or have you not begun the program? Indeed, this is an *attainable* goal, as long as your doctor approves, and this goal is certainly *relevant* to living a long, healthy life. Your goal should be *time based:* you should read this book within five days, buy the equipment you need, and set your exercise schedule within the next five days. Start the program within the following two to three days.

The goals and time frame are entirely up to you. You may want to focus your long-term goals on improving a specific health condition, such as reducing pain from arthritis, controlling diabetes, increasing bone density to help combat osteoporosis, or increasing muscle mass to help with balance or weight control. Or your goal may be to bowl or play tennis, or perhaps to do all of your own chores, such as cleaning windows or vacuuming. Your success depends on setting goals that are truly important to you—and possessing a strong desire to achieve them.

Identifying Your Short-Term Goals
Identify at least two or three of your own short-term goals and write them down. If you have more goals, write them down as well. Remember that each goal should be S-M-A-R-T—specific, measurable, attainable, relevant, and time based. Setting these short-term goals will help motivate you to make the program a regular part of your life.

Examples:

1. I will talk to my doctor about starting this program (if you have any health problems).

2. I will buy the equipment I need and get ready to exercise within two weeks.

3. I will look at my calendar and schedule two or three 45-minute blocks of time for exercise each week.

4. I will invite my spouse/friend/family member to join me in these exercises.

Identifying Your Long-Term Goals
Identify at least two or three long-term goals and write them down. If you have more goals, write them down as well. Are there activities that you want to do more easily over the long term? Are there things that you haven't done in some time that you want to do again? Listing these goals will help you stay with the program, see your progress, and enjoy your success. (Don't forget to use the S-M-A-R-T technique.)

Examples:

1. I will do each exercise two or three times each week. Within three months, I will do each exercise with five-pound weights.

2. After 12 weeks of the program, I will take stairs instead of elevators.

3. I will be able to walk to the store or office.

4. I will do my own vacuuming.

5. I will play golf.

6. I will reduce some of the pain and stiffness from arthritis.

See It and Believe It

I am a firm believer in the mind-body connection in all that we do. Believing in yourself—believing that you can leap barriers and achieve your goals—is the ticket to success. One of the most powerful tools for building self-confidence is visualization. This easy technique involves imagining the accomplishment of the changes or goals you're working to achieve. It is a process of "training" purely within the mind. By visualizing in detail your successful execution of each step of a given activity, you create, modify, or strengthen brain pathways that are important in coordinating your muscles for the visualized activity. This prepares you to perform the activity itself. The technique is useful in many areas of life, from avoiding anxiety during a stressful situation to performing well during competition. You may find it a powerful tool in strength training.

Here is a simple visualization exercise.

1. Identify the goal that you want to visualize—for example, walking an entire golf course.

2. Find a comfortable place to sit and relax.

3. Eliminate all distractions—turn off the phone, television, and so forth.

4. Close your eyes and focus on feeling relaxed. Free your mind of intruding thoughts.

5. Now imagine yourself on the golf course. Create a picture in your mind of the place—the sights, sounds, and smells. Imagine a perfect day, warm and sunny, with a gentle breeze. Picture yourself with your favorite golfing friends, talking and laughing. Now visualize yourself starting on your way, passing the golf carts, and setting off to walk the whole course.

6. Take a moment to feel the pleasure and excitement of achieving this goal.

7. Then imagine yourself walking from hole to hole, enjoying the sunshine, the views, the fresh air, the good company, and the excellent play.

8. Finally, visualize yourself finishing the course and feeling great, both physically and emotionally.

Staying Motivated

No exercise program can succeed if you are bored. Consider these factors that motivate people to begin and stick with exercise programs. Then identify the ones that motivate you.

- Pleasure. People often really enjoy strength-training exercises; they find them less taxing than aerobic workouts and love the results.

- Health and fitness benefits. Strength training increases muscle mass and bone density. It makes you feel strong and energized, alleviates stress and depression, and gives you a better night's sleep. And it can help prevent the onset of certain chronic diseases or ease their symptoms.

- Improvements in appearance. Lifting weights firms the body, trims fat, and can boost metabolism by as much as 15%, which helps with weight control.

■ Social opportunities. Exercising with friends or family gives you a chance to enjoy their company while you work out.

■ Thrills. People who start strength training later in life often find that they are willing and able to try new, exciting activities, such as parasailing, windsurfing, or kayaking.

Tips for a Safe and Successful Physical Activity Program

■ Check with your health-care provider. If you have a chronic health problem such as obesity, diabetes, heart disease, or high blood pressure, ask your health-care provider about what type and amount of physical activity is right for you.

■ Start slowly. Incorporate more physical activity into your daily routine, and gradually work up to 30 to 45 minutes per day. Do not overdo it, as overexercising is actually pro-inflammatory.

■ Set rewards. Celebrate every success—you earned it! Just don't celebrate with a hot fudge sundae.

■ Track your progress. Keep an activity log. Note when you worked out, what activity you did, how long you did the activity, and how you felt during your workout. Also, record the days that you did not work out and what may have caused you to skip exercising.

■ Think variety. Choose a variety of physical activities to help you meet your goals, prevent boredom, and keep your mind and body challenged.

■ Be comfortable. Wear comfortable shoes and clothes that are appropriate to the activity you will be doing.

■ Listen to your body. Stop exercising and consult your health-care provider if you experience chest discomfort or pain, dizziness, severe headache, or other unusual symptoms while you work out. If you have pain that does not go away, get medical help right away. If you are feeling fatigued or sick, take time off from your exercise routine to rest. You can ease back into your program when you start feeling better.

■ Follow the anti-inflammatory, anti-AGEs guidelines of nutritious foods. Choose a variety of these foods every day. Remember that your health and weight depend on both your eating plan and your physical activity level. Healthful foods will give you the energy you need to be active.

■ Get support. Encourage your family and friends to support you and join you in your activity. Form walking groups with coworkers, play with your children outside, or take a dance class with friends.

Equipment Needs

Strength training requires little special equipment, but there are a few basic necessities:

■ *A sturdy chair and exercise space.* Find a strong, stable chair without arms that does not move when you sit in it or when you stand up from it.

When you're seated in the chair, your knees should be at a 90-degree angle, and your feet should be flat on the ground. If the chair is too high, find one with shorter legs; if it's too low, try putting a pillow or a folded blanket on the seat to give you a slight boost.

For your exercise space, choose an open area, preferably carpeted, with at least enough space for your chair and ample room to walk around it. Carpeting will prevent the chair from sliding. On bare floor, put your chair against the wall. If you think you might like to exercise to music or while watching television, plan your space accordingly.

■ *Good shoes.* Good shoes are essential for any outdoor exercise, except swimming, diving, etc. For strength training, try athletic shoes with good support, such as walking, running, or cross-training sneakers. The sole should be rubber, but not too thick, as fat soles may cause you to trip. If you don't already have shoes that fit this description, you can find them at sporting-goods, discount, and department stores.

■ *Comfortable clothing.* Wear loose, cool, comfortable clothing that breathes well during exercise—for example, a cotton T-shirt and cotton shorts or pants. If you want to purchase new workout clothes, look for materials that readily absorb moisture and breathe well.

■ *Dumbbells (hand-held weights) and ankle weights.* You can complete the first part of your exercise program without weights, but as you get stronger and add new exercises, you will need dumbbells and ankle weights. It's a good idea to buy these before you begin strength training, or as soon as possible after you start, so that you'll have them on hand when you're ready to add them to your program. You can also use exercise tubes (also known as resistance bands), which are a great alternative to handheld weights and weight machines. Thanks to some breakthroughs in technology, exercise tubes can be used for a wide range of strength and resistance training. To learn more visit www.exercisetubes.com.

■ Your minimum purchase should include a set of two dumbbells in each of the following weights:

WOMEN	MEN
Two Pounds	Three Pounds
Three Pounds	Five Pounds
Five Pounds	Eight Pounds

The best ankle weights for this program are adjustable weights. These allow you to add weight gradually in increments of a half pound or full pound until you reach as much as 10 or 20 pounds per leg.

Some stores and mail-order companies offer sets of one-pound, three-pound, and five-pound weights at substantial savings. This is a good starter kit; later you can buy heavier dumbbell sets at sporting-goods stores.

■ *Storage container.* For safety reasons, consider storing your weights in a floor-level cupboard or in a container such as a wooden box or canvas bag, preferably on a cart with wheels for easy relocation to your exercise spot. Storage containers and wheeled carts are usually available at local department and discount stores. If you choose not to use a cart, keep your weights in the area where you exercise to minimize transporting them from one area to another. Also, be mindful to store weights out of the reach of children and in a place where people will not trip over them.

Scheduling Exercise

Look at your schedule to see where exercise may best fit in—perhaps on weekday mornings before work or during your favorite evening television program. There are no rules about the best time to exercise. But keep in mind that you should schedule your sessions on three nonconsecutive days of the week (say, Monday, Wednesday, and Friday, or Tuesday, Thursday, and Saturday) in order to give your muscles proper rest. Alternatively, you can do lower body exercises one day and upper body exercises the next; that way, you will avoid overworking the same muscle groups.

Put your scheduled strength-training appointments on your calendar and keep them faithfully, just as you would a doctor's appointment. You can also find an exercise partner who can join you for your scheduled sessions; working with a friend will help you adhere to your regimen and keep you motivated. As Aristotle so succinctly stated, "We are what we repeatedly do." Regular, scheduled exercise is an excellent habit to form. And as Nike says, "Just do it!" This sage advice always works for me.

Here are some tips on scheduling exercise:

■ Consider what days best suit your schedule, given your other commitments.

■ Pick a time of day at which you find exercise enjoyable. Some people like to exercise first thing in the morning; others are more motivated in the afternoon or evening.

- Write your first exercise appointments on your calendar.

- After completing your first two or three sessions, evaluate whether your selected days and times work well for you. If they don't, reexamine your schedule and try to find better times.

Getting Started

The CDC has created an excellent program known as the Growing Stronger Strength Training Program. By joining this program, you will have taken the first step on a journey toward greater strength and vitality. Growing Stronger was designed specifically for those who are new to strength training. It is a great place to start and hopefully progress to a more sophisticated program as your strength and vitality increase—along with sleek, toned, and well-formed muscle mass.

This interactive program is designed to help you build into your life a safe, simple, and highly effective exercise program based on the principles of strength training. Studies at laboratories around the world have shown that strength training benefits women and men of all ages and all levels of fitness. And according to the most recent Surgeon General's report, experts agree that aerobic activities should be supplemented with strength-developing exercises at least twice per week.

The strength-training "prescription" featured here—the motivational tips, safety precautions, and specific exercises—were developed at the exercise research laboratory at Tufts University. Whatever your age, medical condition, or current level of activity, you are likely a perfect candidate for this gentle but powerful regimen of strengthening exercises.

The goal of this program is to help you make strength training a lifelong habit. By so doing, you will be on your way to a strong, independent, and vibrant life!

Warm-up

To get your muscles warm and loose for strength training, walk for 5 to 10 minutes outside if weather permits, or inside around the house or on a treadmill if you have one. Walking will help direct needed blood flow to your muscles, and prepare your body for exercise. Warming up is important for preventing injury as well as gaining maximal benefit from the exercise, because loose, warm muscles will respond better to the challenge of lifting weights. If you have another piece of aerobic exercise equipment, such as an exercise bike, rowing machine, or stair stepper, this will serve as an adequate warm-up as well.

Stage 1

The following four exercises comprise Stage 1 of the Growing Stronger Program. When you've been doing the exercises of this stage for at least two weeks, *or* if you are fairly fit right now, you can add the exercises in Stage 2. Remember to always do the Warm-up and Cooldown (see pages 263 and 272) as part of each exercise session.

Squats: This is a great exercise for strengthening hips, thighs, and buttocks. Before long, you'll find that walking, jogging, and climbing stairs are a snap!

1. Standing with your back in front of the seat a sturdy, armless chair, plant your feet slightly more than shoulder-width apart. Extend your arms so they are parallel to the ground, and keep your torso straight up and down.

2. Making sure that your knees *never* come forward past your toes, lower yourself in a slow, controlled motion, to a count of four, until you are almost sitting on the seat of the chair.

3. Pause. Then, to a count of two, slowly rise back to a standing position. Keep your knees over your ankles and your back straight.

4. Repeat 10 times for one set. Rest for one to two minutes. Then complete a second set of 10 repetitions.

Note: If this exercise is too difficult, start off by using your hands for assistance. If you are unable to go all the way down, place a couple of pillows on the chair or only lower yourself four to six inches.

MAKE SURE YOU:

- Don't sit down too quickly.

- Don't lean your weight too far forward or onto your toes when standing up.

Wall Push-ups: This exercise is a modified version of the push-up you may have done years ago in physical education classes. It is less challenging than a classic push-up and won't require you to get down on the floor—but it will help strengthen and tone your arms, shoulders, and chest.

1. Find a wall that is clear of any objects. Stand a little farther than arm's length from the wall.

2. Facing the wall, lean your body forward and place your palms flat against the wall at about shoulder height and shoulder-width apart. Inhale.

3. To a count of four, bend your elbows as you lower your upper body toward the wall in a slow, controlled motion, keeping your feet planted. Exhale as you move forward.

4. Pause. Then, to a count of two, slowly push yourself back until your arms are straight—but don't lock your elbows. Inhale as you return to starting position.

5. Repeat 10 times for one set. Rest for one to two minutes. Then complete a second set of 10 repetitions.

MAKE SURE YOU:

- Don't round or arch your back.

Toe Stands: This is a good way to strengthen your calves and ankles and restore stability and balance.

1. Near a counter or sturdy chair, stand with feet shoulder-width apart. Use the back of the chair or a counter for balance. Inhale.

2. To a count of four, slowly rise as far as you can onto the balls of your feet and hold for two to four seconds. This is a ballet relevé. Exhale as you rise.

3. Then, to a count of four, slowly lower your heels back to the floor. Inhale as you lower.

4. Repeat 10 times for one set. Rest for one to two minutes. Then complete a second set of 10 repetitions.

MAKE SURE YOU:

■ Don't lean on the counter or chair—use it for balance only.

Finger Marching: In this exercise you'll let your fingers, hands, and arms do the walking. This will help strengthen your upper body and your grip, and increase the flexibility of your arms, back, and shoulders.

1. Stand, or sit in an armless chair, with your feet on the floor, shoulder-width apart.

2. Movement 1: Imagine that there is a wall directly in front of you. Slowly walk your fingers up the wall until your arms are above your head. Hold them overhead while wiggling your fingers for about 10 seconds and then slowly walk them back down.

3. Movement 2: Next, try to touch your two hands behind your back. If you can, reach for the opposite elbow with each hand—or get as close as you can. Hold the position for about 10 seconds, feeling a stretch in the back, arms, and chest.

4. Movement 3: Release your arms and finger-weave your hands in front of your body. Raise your arms so that they're parallel to the ground, with your palms facing the imaginary wall. Sit or stand up straight, but curl your shoulders forward. You should feel the stretch in your wrist and upper back. Hold the position for about 10 seconds.

5. Repeat this three-part exercise three times.

Stage 2

When you've been doing the exercises from Stage 1 for at least two weeks, *or* if you are fairly fit right now, you can add these four Stage 2 exercises. When you've been doing the exercises from Stages 1 and 2 for at least six weeks, you can add the exercises in Stage 3. Remember to always do the Warm-up and Cooldown as part of each exercise session.

Biceps Curl: This exercise will quickly increase your arm strength, enabling you to lift heavier objects without strain or discomfort.

1. With a 3 lb. or 5 lb. dumbbell in each hand, stand or sit in an armless chair, with feet shoulder-width apart, arms at your sides, and palms facing your thighs.

2. To a count of two, slowly lift the weights so that your forearms rotate and palms face in toward your shoulders, while keeping your upper arms and elbows close to your sides—as if you had a newspaper tucked beneath your arm. Keep your wrists straight and dumbbells parallel to the floor. Exhale as you lift.

3. Pause. Then, to a count of four, slowly lower the dumbbells back toward your thighs, rotating your forearms so that your arms are again at your sides, with your palms facing your thighs. Inhale as you lower.

4. Repeat 10 times for one set. Rest for one to two minutes. Then complete a second set of 10 repetitions.

MAKE SURE YOU:

- Don't let your elbows move away from the sides of your body.

- Keep your wrists straight.

Step-Ups: This is a great strengthening exercise that requires only a set of stairs or some aerobic "steps." But don't let its simplicity fool you. Step-ups will improve your balance and build strength in your legs, hips, and buttocks.

1. Stand alongside the handrail at the bottom of a staircase (or stand behind your small aerobic steps). With your feet flat and toes facing forward, put your right foot on the first step.

2. Holding the handrail for balance, to a count of two, straighten your right leg to lift your left leg slowly until it reaches the first step. As you're lifting yourself, make sure that your right knee stays straight and does not move forward past your ankle. Let your left foot tap the first step near your right foot.

3. Pause. Then, using your right leg to support your weight, to a count of four, slowly lower your left foot back to the floor.

4. Repeat 10 times with the right leg and 10 times with the left leg for one set. Rest for one to two minutes. Then complete a second set of 10 repetitions with each leg.

MAKE SURE YOU:

▪ Don't let your back leg do the work.

▪ Don't let momentum do the work.

▪ Your weight should be evenly distributed throughout the standing foot (the right foot in steps 1–4 above).

▪ Breathe normally throughout this exercise.

Overhead Press: This useful exercise targets several muscles in the arms, upper back, and shoulders. It can also help firm the back of your upper arms, and make reaching for objects in high cupboards easier.

1. Stand, or sit in an armless chair, with feet shoulder-width apart, and arms at your sides, palms facing forward. With a dumbbell in each hand, raise your hands, palms facing forward, until the dumbbells are level with your shoulders and parallel to the floor. Inhale.

2. To a count of two, slowly push the dumbbells up over your head until your arms are fully extended—but don't lock your elbows. Exhale as you lift.

3. Pause. Then, to a count of four, slowly lower the dumbbells back to your sides, bringing your elbows down close to your sides. Inhale as you lower.

4. Repeat 10 times for one set. Rest for one to two minutes. Then complete a second set of 10 repetitions.

MAKE SURE YOU:

■ Keep your wrists straight.

■ Don't lock your elbows.

■ Don't let the dumbbells move too far in front of your body or behind it.

Hip Abduction: By targeting the muscles of the hips, thighs, and buttocks, this exercise makes your lower body shapelier, and strengthens your hipbones, which may be especially vulnerable to fracture as you age.

1. Stand behind a sturdy chair, with feet slightly apart and toes facing forward. Keep your legs straight, but do not lock your knees. Inhale.

2. To a count of two, slowly lift your right leg out to the side. Keep your left leg straight—but again, do not lock your knee. Exhale as you lift.

3. Pause. Then, to a count of four, slowly lower your right foot back to the ground. Inhale as you lower.

4. Repeat 10 times with the right leg and 10 times with the left leg for one set. Rest for one to two minutes. Then complete a second set of 10 repetitions with each leg. To increase the difficulty of this exercise, you may add ankle weights.

MAKE SURE YOU:

■ Don't lock your knee on the supporting leg.

■ Keep your toes facing forward throughout the move.

■ Don't lean to the side when you lift your leg.

Stage 3

When you've been doing the exercises from Stage 1 and Stage 2 for at least six weeks, you can add these four Stage 3 exercises. Remember to always do the Warm-up and Cooldown as part of each exercise session.

Knee Extension: By targeting the quadriceps muscles in the front of the thigh (which play a primary role in bending and straightening the leg), this exercise strengthens weak knees, and reduces the symptoms of arthritis of the knee. It is important to do this exercise in conjunction with the next exercise, the knee curl, as the muscles targeted in these two exercises—the front thigh muscles and the hamstrings—work together when you walk, stand, and climb.

1. Put on your ankle weights.

2. In a sturdy, armless chair, sit all the way back, so that your feet barely touch the ground; this will allow for easier movement throughout the exercise. If your chair is too low, add a rolled-up towel under your knees. Your feet should be shoulder-width apart, and your arms should rest at your sides or on your thighs. Inhale.

3. With your toes pointing forward and your foot flexed, to a count of two slowly lift your right leg, extending your leg until your knee is straight. Exhale as you lift.

4. Pause. Then, to a count of four, slowly lower your foot back to the ground. Inhale as you lower.

5. Repeat 10 times with the right leg and 10 times with the left leg for one set. Rest for a minute or two. Then complete a second set of 10 repetitions with each leg.

MAKE SURE YOU:

▪ Keep your ankle flexed throughout the move.

Knee Curl: This is an excellent exercise for strengthening the muscles of the back of the upper leg, known as the hamstrings. When done in conjunction with the knee extension, it makes walking and climbing easier.

1. Put on your ankle weights.

2. Stand behind a sturdy chair, with feet shoulder-width apart and facing forward.

3. Keeping your foot flexed, to a count of two slowly bend your right leg, bringing your heel up toward your buttocks.

4. Pause. Then, to a count of four, slowly lower your foot back to the ground.

5. Repeat 10 times with your right leg and 10 times with your left leg for one set. Rest for a minute or two. Then complete a second set of 10 repetitions with each leg.

MAKE SURE YOU:

■ Keep the thigh of the bending leg in line with the supporting leg at all times.

■ Keep the foot on the bending leg flexed throughout the move.

■ Breathe normally throughout this exercise.

Pelvic Tilt: This exercise improves posture and tightens the muscles in your abdomen and buttocks. Do this exercise in conjunction with the next exercise, the floor back extension, to strengthen your midsection. (You should not have the ankle weights on during this exercise.)

1. On the floor or on a firm mattress, lie flat on your back with your knees bent, feet flat on the floor or mattress, and arms at your sides, palms facing the ground. Inhale.

2. To a count of two, slowly roll your pelvis so that your hips and lower back are off the floor, while your upper back and shoulders remain in place. Exhale as you lift.

3. Pause. Then, to a count of four, slowly lower your pelvis all the way down. Inhale as you lower.

4. Repeat 10 times for one set. Rest for a minute or two. Then complete a second set of 10 repetitions.

MAKE SURE YOU:

■ Don't lift your upper back or shoulders off the ground.

Floor Back Extension: If you suffer from lower back pain, weak abdominal muscles may be to blame. The floor back extension, done in conjunction with the pelvic tilt, will strengthen these muscles and ease back pain.

1. Lie facedown on the floor, with a pillow under your hips. Extend your arms straight overhead on the floor.

2. To a count of two, slowly lift your right arm and left leg off the floor, keeping them at the same level. Your foot should be stretched, and your leg should be straight, but don't lock your knee. Inhale as you lift.

3. Pause. Then, to a count of four, slowly lower your arm and leg back to the floor. Exhale as you lower.

4. Repeat 10 times for one set, and then switch to left arm with right leg for a set of 10 repetitions.

5. Rest for a minute or two. Then complete a second set of 10 repetitions with each leg.

MAKE SURE YOU:

■ Keep your head, neck, and back in a straight line. Don't lift your head more than an inch or two off of the floor.

Cooldown

Quadriceps Stretch: This excellent stretch should be a regular part of your cooldown. Strength-training exercises such as squats, step-ups, and knee extensions focus on strengthening the quadriceps muscles. This stretch will help these muscles relax, and make them more flexible.

1. Stand next to a counter or sturdy chair with your feet about shoulder-width apart and your knees straight, but not locked.

2. With your left hand, hold a chair or counter for balance. Bend your

right leg back and grasp your right ankle in your right hand until your thigh is perpendicular to the ground. Make sure you stand up straight—don't lean forward. (If you can't grasp your ankle in your hand, just keep your leg as close to perpendicular as possible and hold the bend, or place your foot on the seat of a chair.) You should feel a stretch in the front of the thigh.

3. Hold the stretch for a slow count of 30 to 40, breathing throughout.

4. Release your right ankle and repeat with the other leg.

MAKE SURE YOU:

■ Breathe throughout the stretch, concentrating on relaxing.

■ Stand up straight and look straight ahead.

■ Don't lock your supporting knee.

Hamstring/Calf Stretch: If touching your toes with straight legs seems an impossible task, you're not alone. Many people have tight hamstring and calf muscles in the backs of their legs. This stretch will give these muscles more flexibility and make it easier for you to bend over.

1. Sit in a chair with your knees bent and your feet flat on the floor.

2. Extend your right leg in front of you, placing your right heel on the floor, and keeping your ankle relaxed. Don't lock your knee. Inhale. Exhale as you slowly lean forward at the hips, bending toward your right toes, trying to keep your back straight. Stretch your right foot as you stretch forward.

3. Hold the stretch for a slow count of 20 to 30, breathing throughout.

4. Sit up straight again and flex your right ankle so that your toes are pointing up toward the ceiling. Again, inhale, then exhale as you lean forward at the hips, bending toward your right toes, and hold the stretch for a slow count of 20 to 30, breathing throughout.

5. Release the stretch and repeat with your left leg.

Note: You should feel the first part of this stretch in the back of the upper leg and the second part in the calf.

MAKE SURE YOU:

▪ Keep your back straight and head lifted as you lean forward toward your toes.

▪ Don't push the stretch too far—it shouldn't be painful.

Chest and Arm Stretch: This simple reaching stretch will improve the flexibility in your arms and chest and in the front of your shoulders.

1. Stand with your arms at your sides and your feet about shoulder-width apart. Inhale.

2. Extend both arms behind your back and clasp your hands together, if possible, retracting your shoulders. Exhale.

3. Hold the stretch for a slow count of 20 to 30, breathing throughout.

4. Inhale as you release the stretch and repeat.

MAKE SURE YOU:

▪ Breathe throughout the stretch.

▪ Keep your back straight and look straight ahead.

Neck, Upper Back, and Shoulder Stretch: This easy stretch targets another group of muscles particularly vulnerable to tension and stress—the neck, back, and shoulders. Do it often—after strength training, and during any activity that makes you feel stiff, such as sitting at a desk or at a computer. You'll find it rejuvenating.

1. Stand with your feet shoulder-width apart, your knees straight but not locked, and your hands clasped in front of you.

2. Rotate your hands so that your palms are facing the ground; then raise your arms to about chest height. Inhale.

3. Gently press your palms away from your body. You should feel a stretch in your neck and upper back and along your shoulders. Exhale as you press.

4. Hold the stretch for a slow count of 20 to 30, breathing throughout.

5. Inhale as you release the stretch and repeat.

MAKE SURE YOU:

- Breathe throughout the stretch.

- Don't curve your back or arch it.

More Exercises

The following five exercises can be added to your routine after you are comfortable doing the Stage 3 exercises.

Abdominal Curl: The abdominal muscles provide bracing and stability to the trunk, especially the lower back. Strengthening this group of muscles can help your posture, and prevent back pain.

1. Lie on your back on the floor, knees bent, and feet flat on the floor.

2. Place your hands behind your head, elbows pointing out. Inhale.

3. Exhale as you slowly raise your shoulders and upper back off of the floor to the count of two.

4. Pause. Inhale as you slowly lower your shoulders back to the floor to the count of two.

5. Repeat 10 times for one set. Rest for one to two minutes. Then complete a second set.

MAKE SURE YOU:

- Don't pull on your head or neck with your hands.

- Keep your chin lifted toward the ceiling and elbows pointed out throughout the exercise.

Chest Press: This exercise targets the muscles of the chest and shoulders.

1. Lie on your back on the floor, knees bent, and feet flat on the floor.

2. Hold a dumbbell in each hand at chest level, about shoulder-width apart. Your elbows should be bent and your palms should face your knees. Inhale.

3. Exhale as you slowly straighten your arms toward the ceiling, directly above your chest, to a count of two.

4. Pause. Inhale as you slowly lower the dumbbells back to your chest, to a count of four.

5. Repeat 10 times for one set. Rest for one to two minutes. Then complete a second set.

MAKE SURE YOU:

■ Raise the dumbbells directly above your chest. Don't let your arms move toward your head or your waist as you lift.

Lunge: The lunge strengthens the muscles of the upper leg and hips.

1. Stand beside (not facing) a counter or sturdy chair with your feet about shoulder-width apart. Hold the counter or chair with your right hand for balance. Inhale.

2. Exhale and take a large step forward with your right foot.

3. Bend your right knee and lower your hips toward the floor. Make sure that your right knee stays above your right ankle as you lower. Keep left leg straight, foot on floor.

4. Push against the floor with your right foot to raise yourself, and step back to the starting position. Inhale as you step back.

5. Repeat 10 times with your right leg for one set.

6. Rest for one to two minutes. Then repeat with your left leg.

■ Don't allow your front knee to move forward past your toes.

■ Keep your upper body straight and erect during the exercise. Don't lean forward or backward.

■ Try to lower your hips until your front thigh is parallel to the floor. If that's too difficult, just lower as far as you can.

Upright Row: This exercise strengthens upper arms and upper back muscles.

1. Stand with feet about hip-width apart, holding a dumbbell in each hand.

2. Hold the dumbbells in front of your thighs, palms facing your thighs. Inhale.

3. Exhale as you bend your elbows and raise the dumbbells in front of your body, to the count of two, until they are at shoulder height.

4. Pause. Inhale as you lower the dumbbells, to the count of four, to the starting position.

5. Repeat 10 times for one set. Rest for one to two minutes, then complete a second set.

■ Keep your back straight throughout the exercise.

Gaining Grip Strength: If you have arthritis, you may have trouble picking things up with your hands or keeping a grip on them. Some of the exercises in this program will help strengthen your hand muscles. If you're concerned about grip strength, you may also want to add a grip exercise to increase strength and decrease stiffness in your hands. The exercise is simple; it can be done easily while reading or watching TV, and most people already have the equipment at home.

■ Equipment: Racquetball, tennis ball, or "stress" ball.

■ Time: Less than 5 minutes.

■ Exercise: Grasp a ball in one hand while sitting or standing. Slowly squeeze it as hard as you can and hold the squeeze for three to five seconds. Slowly release the squeeze. Take a short rest, then repeat the exercise 10 times. Switch hands, and do two sets of 10 squeezes with the other hand.

■ Frequency: You may do this exercise every day or every other day, depending on how your hands feel. If they feel stiff or painful, you may want to skip a day.

Frequently Asked Questions

1. Can the Growing Stronger Exercise Program be done three times a week if I have the time? What about just once a week when I'm really busy?

New guidelines from the American College of Sports Medicine suggest strength training two or three times a week. Be sure to give your muscles at least one day of rest between workouts. Two sessions are prescribed because this will confer benefits. Two sessions per week are also quite manageable from a time perspective. However, if you have the time to do the program three times per week, you will gain the following benefits:

■ More stimuli to the bones

■ Extra physical activity—important for overall good health

■ Strengthening muscles a bit more quickly

If you do decide to do the program three times per week, just make sure they are on nonconsecutive days, such as Monday, Wednesday, and Friday. If you can only do the program one day per week when your schedule gets hectic, that is certainly better than nothing. But we recommend that you try to get in two days per week whenever possible.

2. When I do the knee extension to a full stretch, even with minimal weight, my knees make the most awful noises and also hurt (with sharp pains). If I don't go all the way, my knees are noisy but don't hurt. So should I persevere with the full stretch, or would I be better off not trying to stretch completely?

First, you should discuss your knee symptoms with your physician and follow his or her recommendations. In the meantime, you might do the exercises with reduced weight (or no weight) and through a reduced range of motion—whatever it takes for you to do the exercises without pain. Don't worry about the noises, but do avoid pain. Then progress slowly, cautiously increasing both the range of motion and the amount of weight you're lifting. Over time, you should be able to strengthen your legs and improve your flexibility.

3. Why can't I make my own weights for working out?

Many suggestions exist for homemade weights, ranging from lifting one-pound soup cans (harmless for you and the soup, but it won't build muscle), to lifting buckets or gallon jugs filled with sand. Please do not improvise! Plastic buckets and jugs are not made for strength training; they're not designed to hold that much weight, and the handles are designed for carrying, not lifting. They could easily break and injure you, not to mention impede your ability to perform an exercise with proper form and through the full range of motion.

4. Is it true that muscle weighs more than fat? If so, will I gain weight when I start strength training if I don't go on a diet?

Unless you increase the amount of calories you are eating, it is very unlikely that you will gain weight or become bulky. Here's why. One pound equals one pound regardless of whether the pound is fat, muscle, or some other substance like butter or steel. Muscle is denser, and therefore takes up a smaller amount of space per pound than fat. Some scientists estimate that the "space" that one pound of muscle occupies is about 22% less than one pound of fat! If you begin strength training and continue to eat the

same number of calories, you may lose some weight because you're burning additional calories while exercising. The important thing about
strength training is the change in body composition. You will gain muscle
and most likely decrease body fat even if your body weight stays the same.
In our experience, people might drop a size or two after they have been
strength training for a couple of months because their body shape has
changed for the better. If your goal in starting strength training is to gain
weight, we recommend that you also increase the number of calories you
are consuming. Try adding an extra fruit, vegetable, low-fat dairy, and/or
whole-grain serving to your daily diet.

5. What is the proper way to breathe during strength training?

Exhale during the most-strenuous phase of the movement—often referred to as "exhale on the exertion." Inhale during the less-strenuous
phase. It is also important to inhale and exhale fully between each repetition.

    However, the most important thing is to simply breathe regularly. Most
people assume that they are automatically breathing when they are actually holding their breath. Take a moment to focus on your breathing during your next strength-training session and during other strenuous
activities such as climbing stairs. You may be surprised to find that you
are actually holding your breath.

6. I have a medical condition. Can I still do strength training?

Most likely you will be able to participate in strength training; however,
this is a decision you must make in consultation with your doctor or
health-care provider. Discuss your specific conditions and goals with
your physician so that he or she can make any necessary recommendations.

    Research has shown that individuals with chronic but stable medical
conditions, including osteoporosis, heart disease, diabetes, rheumatoid
arthritis, osteoarthritis, and HIV/AIDS, and the frail elderly, can benefit
significantly from strength training.

It is important to start conservatively and progress slowly. Consider working with a qualified fitness instructor, at least for a few sessions, to make sure your exercise form is correct. Pay attention to your body. Strength training should never cause pain. Feeling good is an indication that you are exercising properly.

To learn more, log on to www.cdc.gov, which is a veritable gold mine on all forms of physical exercise.

In our next chapter you will learn how to prepare delicious recipes that won't promote the formation of age-accelerating AGEs.

11

AGE-less Recipes

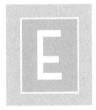njoying great food is one of life's pleasures. Fortunately, there are many foods and many outstanding ways to prepare them that will not accelerate the aging process, ruin your skin, and/or pack on unwanted pounds. As always, foods that are lower on the glycemic index are much more preferable than foods that are higher. Controlling blood sugar and insulin levels is not only critical to slowing down aging and preventing weight gain, but is important in preventing the formation of AGEs.

Important Tips to Remember

- Always start your meal with protein. This will help suppress your appetite and prevent overeating. Protein is neutral when it comes to pro-inflammatory foods versus anti-inflammatory foods. This means that it will not raise your blood-sugar or insulin level and promote AGE formation. Remember, though, that if you eat protein that has been breaded and fried, this changes the equation.

▪ If you want to enjoy a piece of fish or chicken that does have breading on it, use ground nuts or seeds (assuming that you have no allergies) or ground oats. This works very well, has a healthy fat component, and adds great flavor.

▪ Don't go fat free unless you want dry skin, brittle hair and nails, depression, lack of energy, and fading memory and brain power. Fats provide us with the all-important building blocks for cell membranes, hormones, and prostaglandins, which act as regulators throughout the body. Fats also function as carriers for fat-soluble vitamins, including vitamins A, D, E, and K. Dietary fats are also necessary to convert carotene to vitamin A, and for a host of other processes.

▪ If you like to eat an occasional meal of red meat, try to purchase grass-fed meat as opposed to grain-fed meat. It has a much healthier fatty-acid profile, and is a good source of conjugated linoleic acid.

▪ Just three small apples a day will help control your weight, stabilize blood sugar, and provide antioxidants and fiber.

▪ More good news about apples and fish—a study performed at Utrecht University in the Netherlands found that the children of mothers who consumed the highest amount of apples while pregnant had significantly fewer asthma symptoms than the children of mothers who consumed the least amount of apples. Interestingly, the researchers found no such comparable benefit from juice or other fruit consumption. The same researchers also found that the children of mothers who ate fish at least once or more per week had significantly fewer incidences of eczema (an inflammatory skin condition that causes areas of the skin to become red, itchy, and scaly) than the children of mothers who did not eat fish. Researchers concluded that it was the antioxidant flavonoids in the apples that prevented the asthma, and the essential fatty acids in the fish that prevented the eczema. Cold-water fish such as salmon, sardines, herring, trout, and anchovies are the best sources of essential fatty acids in fish.

- Don't forget the fiber—beans and lentils are great sources. Try adding a couple of tablespoons of chickpeas to your salads.

- Beans and lentils will also exert blood sugar–stabilizing effects for many hours—try to include them at lunch and dinner.

- Use fresh and dried spices and herbs often—these pungent power-houses truly are the fountain of youth—from cinnamon to turmeric, oregano to ginger.

- Drink six to eight glasses of pure spring water per day—especially as you increase your fiber intake.

- Give up coffee—it can increase stress, and roasted coffee beans can be a source of exogenous AGEs. Even decaf coffee beans have been roasted, so they too can be a source of AGEs.

- Choose organic, free-range chicken and turkey for superior flavor and to avoid the antibiotics and processing of regular commercially raised poultry.

- Choose eggs from cage-free chickens that are fed diets high in the omega-3s, such as flaxseed. These eggs are now widely available, and are a much healthier choice than conventional eggs.

- Buy organic. Pesticides can leave toxic residues on plants that can harm your organ systems.

- Anchovies can increase skin firmness and radiance. Mash up one or two and add them to salad dressings. This is the secret of the famous Caesar salad dressing.

- Sauté foods over medium heat, and remember to not brown the foods—proteins or vegetables.

- Enjoy a yogurt or kefir smoothie as a morning and/or afternoon snack. Add SuperBerry Powder or Pom Wonderful pomegranate juice, or a tablespoon or two of green foods such as Green Magma Plus or Veggie Magma introduced in Chapter 3. This will give you the all-important probiotics, antioxidants, and anti-AGEs ingredients in one delicious beverage.

- Use garnishes to add flavor and nutrients to each dish. Superior garnishes include chopped organic raw unsalted nuts and seeds; fresh herbs; chives, scallions, green onions, and other tasty snippets from the onion family; and all types of sprouts, especially broccoli sprouts.

- For extra protein, add hard-boiled omega-3 eggs to salads.

- Buy organic citrus. This will enable you to use the zest of the fruit in many recipes, adding bioflavonoids and great taste.

- More reasons to drink green tea or take green-tea supplements—a new study led by Dr. Michael B. Chancellor, professor of urology and gynecology at the University of Pittsburgh School of Medicine, found that the catechins in green tea could be a treatment option for various bladder conditions that are caused by injury or inflammation.

The recipes* in this chapter are courtesy of Wild Oats Markets (www .wildoats.com), a one-stop supermarket for natural and organic foods. Wild Oats is a national chain of full-service supermarkets offering a complete selection of the highest-quality natural and organic food; helpful supplements; and gentle, environmentally friendly household and body-care products. They also offer a gourmet deli filled with many delicious items to grab on the go, as well as full-service seafood, other meat, bakery, floral, and food-service departments. This is a great convenience if you want to enjoy a healthy lunch or dinner but are pressed for time. Wild Oats' rigorous criteria for product selection meet the highest standards in the natural-foods industry. Because of this they carry products that do not contain any hydrogenated oils or artificial colors, flavors, or preservatives.

To find a Wild Oats Market near you and to find additional healthy, fabulous recipes, visit www.wildoats.com.

*A special note on these recipes: Tofu can be substituted in any recipe calling for fish or poultry.

MARINADES

As we have learned, marinating foods, and thereby infusing them with liquids, helps prevent the formation of AGEs during the cooking process. Just remember to use gentle heat. These versatile marinades lend themselves to seafood, poultry, other meats, tofu, and vegetables.

USE-IT-ON-EVERYTHING MARINADE

This delicious marinade works well on virtually everything—from veggies and fish to poultry and steak. Look for grass-fed beef.

PREP TIME: 15 minutes. **MARINATE TIME:** overnight. Makes enough for 20 lbs (about 5½ cups) of fish, tofu, poultry, veggies, etc.

1 red onion, sliced	3 tsp. basil
1 bulb garlic, crushed	4 tsp. Worcestershire sauce
4 tsp. each salt and white pepper	1 cup lemon juice
4 tsp. black pepper	⅓ quart red wine vinegar
4 tsp. paprika	1 quart organic olive oil

Mix all ingredients until well blended. Pour over fish, poultry, etc. and let marinate overnight.

FRAMBOISE MARINADE

3 cups fresh or frozen raspberries	2 bay leaves
½ cup cider vinegar	1 tbsp. dried thyme
½ cup framboise (raspberry liquer)	Salt and freshly ground black pepper
¾ cup olive oil	to taste

Combine raspberries, vinegar, and framboise in saucepan. Heat to just before boiling. Remove from heat. Stir in olive oil, bay leaves, and thyme. Cool to room temperature.

Pour over chicken and sprinkle with salt and pepper. Marinate overnight in refrigerator.

RED ZIN, DIJON, FRESH HERB, AND ROASTED GARLIC MARINADE

2 cups red zinfandel

2 tbsp. organic extra-virgin olive oil

1 tbsp. organic Dijon mustard

1 bulb roasted garlic cloves

3 sprigs rosemary, leaves only

2 sprigs thyme, leaves only

1 tsp. dry basil

Place wine, oil, mustard, garlic cloves, rosemary, thyme leaves, and basil in blender or food processor. Pulse to mix well. Pour over steaks and marinate in the refrigerator for at least one hour, up to six hours.

FRESH TOMATO SALSA

PREP TIME: 20 minutes. **YIELDS:** 3 cups.

6 tomatoes, diced small

2 oz. fresh basil leaves, shredded

4 cloves fresh garlic, minced

¼ cup organic olive oil

1 tsp. kosher salt

1½ tsp. ground black pepper

Wash and dice tomatoes. Place into a mixing bowl and combine with the fresh basil, garlic, oil, salt, and pepper. Toss to coat. Marinate for 15 minutes prior to using. Mixture can also be refrigerated.

ZESTY COCKTAIL SAUCE

PREP TIME: 5 minutes. **CHILL TIME:** 1 hour. Serves 4-6.

¾ cup unsweetened ketchup

1 tbsp. lemon juice (or vinegar)

1 tbsp. prepared horseradish

½ tsp. Worcestershire sauce

4 drops cayenne pepper sauce
(one brand is Texas Champagne®)

Mix all ingredients well and chill thoroughly before serving.

THE MAIN COURSE

These delightful recipes employ gentle cooking methods and provide AGE-defying antioxidant benefits in addition to exceptional flavor. Vegetarians will discover that they can substitute firm tofu for the poultry or seafood in many of these recipes with rewarding results.

Seafood

ALASKAN HALIBUT WITH STRAWBERRY, TANGERINE, & FRESH BASIL SALSA

Fresh, tender halibut combined with tangy strawberry and tangerine and a touch of fresh basil. Serve with a green salad or vegetable.

PREP TIME: 15 minutes. **COOKING TIME:** 15 minutes. Serves 4.

4 8-oz. Alaskan halibut fillets	3 fresh tangerines, peeled, seeded, diced medium
kosher salt, to taste	
black pepper, to taste	1 tbsp. fresh basil, shredded
	½ tsp. balsamic vinegar
FOR SALSA:	
16 oz organic strawberries, hulled, diced medium	⅛ tsp. cayenne pepper
	¼ tsp. kosher salt

Combine the strawberries, tangerines, basil, vinegar, pepper, and salt in a mixing bowl. Toss to completely mix, and marinate for 30 minutes prior to using.

Preheat an oven to 300° F. Season the fish lightly with salt and pepper and grill over medium heat, or prepare in the oven. Remove the cooked fish, arrange on dinner plates or serving platter, and ribbon the salsa over the top of the fish.

BAKED HALIBUT FILLETS WITH FRESH VEGETABLES

When you want a light, yet still filling meal, try this easy recipe. Serve with a twist of lemon to accent the naturally good taste of fresh halibut.

PREP TIME: 15 minutes, plus time to marinate. **COOKING TIME:** 15 minutes. Serves 4.

1 tsp. organic olive oil	2 tbsp. fresh basil, chopped
1 cup diced organic zucchini	¼ tsp. salt
½ cup minced organic onion	¼ tsp. ground black pepper
1 clove garlic, peeled and minced	4 halibut fillets, about 6 oz. each
2 cups diced fresh organic tomatoes	⅓ cup feta cheese, crumbled

Preheat oven to 450° F. Lightly grease a medium baking dish or spray with vegetable oil.

In a medium saucepan, heat olive oil over medium heat and stir in zucchini, onion, and garlic. Sauté lightly for about 5 minutes, or until tender. Turn off heat and mix in tomatoes, basil, salt, and pepper.

Arrange halibut steaks in the baking dish. Top each fillet with an equal amount of the zucchini mixture and sprinkle with feta cheese. Bake 15 minutes, or until fillets flake easily with a fork.

CITRUS-GRILLED SALMON

Delicious with a crisp, green salad.

PREP TIME: 15 minutes, plus time to marinate. Serves 4

1 cup natural orange juice	½ tsp. yellow mustard seed
¼ cup tamari or soy sauce	salt and pepper to taste
2 cloves garlic, minced	4 (6-oz.) salmon fillets
1 tbsp. minced ginger	3 tbsp. diced green onions
1 tsp. organic Dijon mustard	canola oil

Mix together orange juice, tamari, garlic, ginger, mustard, and mustard seed in a glass baking dish. Add salmon, seasoned with salt and pepper, cover, and refrigerate 1 to 4 hours, turning salmon once or twice.

Heat grill or grill pan over medium-high heat. Brush grate or pan lightly with canola oil. Place salmon on grill. Cook 5 minutes each side, per inch of thickness. Let salmon rest 3 minutes before serving. Garnish with green onions.

WHOLE BAKED SALMON
WITH SMOKY BACON, LEMON, AND DILL

TOTAL TIME: 1 hour and 10 minutes. Serves 6.

1 6 lb. whole salmon, cleaned	6 dill sprigs
salt and pepper to taste	1 lemon, sliced into 8 rounds
6 strips nitrate-free bacon, uncooked (Wild Oats, Coleman)	2 cloves garlic, thinly sliced
	¼ cup olive oil

Preheat oven to 325° F. Rinse salmon and pat dry. Season inside of salmon with salt and pepper. Place bacon, dill, lemon, and garlic inside salmon. Rub salmon skin with olive oil and season with salt and pepper. Wrap salmon in foil and place on a baking sheet. Bake for 1 hour. Allow to cool 10 minutes. Remove foil and carefully remove salmon skin and discard bacon, dill, lemon, and garlic. Remove top fillet. Place on a cutting board. Carefully remove the bones. Place remaining fillet on cutting board. Remove any extra skin. Portion into fillets.

ATLANTIC COD WITH SZECHUAN PEPPERCORNS

Recipe provided by Bonny Doon Vineyards, courtesy of Wild Oats

PREP TIME: 20 minutes plus; time to marinade. Serves 4.

2 tbsp. coarse salt	¾ cup fish stock
2 lbs. Atlantic cod fillet	4 tbsp. extra-virgin olive oil
2 tbsp. Szechuan peppercorns	juice of ½ lemon
3 tbsp. pink peppercorns	2 tbsp. unsalted butter
2 bunches baby spinach	salt

The day before, sprinkle the salt over the cod fillet and place on a rack over a rimmed baking sheet. Cover and refrigerate overnight.

Rinse fish and cut into 4 portions. Coarsely grind the peppercorns and sprinkle over the entire cod.

Pour the fish stock into a sauté pan, bring to a boil, and whisk in 3 tbsp. of olive oil slowly. Season and finish with lemon juice.

Sauté fish in 1 tbsp. of olive oil and butter until done. Remove from pan and sauté the spinach, turning every ten seconds or so, for about a minute. Place ¼ of the cooked spinach in the center of each plate, add the piece of cod, and drizzle the olive oil emulsion over the fish. Serve immediately.

CEVICHE

If you've ever treated yourself to a balmy beach vacation in the Yucatán peninsula, this fresh, light, and cool seafood salad will transport you back to paradise. A traditional dish of Peru, as well as a favorite in coastal towns in Mexico and Ecuador, this seafood salad is traditionally "cooked" in lime juice. The acid in the lime juice breaks down the protein in the fish, resulting in a firm, cooked texture. We opted to poach our version to ensure food safety and reduce cooking time.

PREP TIME: 15 minutes plus time to chill. **COOKING TIME:** 10 minutes. Serves 6.

3 cups water or chicken broth

¼ cup white wine

juice of two limes

1 jalapeño or Serrano chili sliced in half

3 cloves garlic, crushed

½ lb. firm white fish fillet (halibut)

½ lb. large shrimp, peeled and
   deveined

2 large, ripe organic tomatoes

½ organic white onion

1 jalapeño, seeded and diced

juice of two limes

¼ cup cilantro, diced

hot sauce to taste

sea salt and cracked black pepper to
   taste

Bring broth, wine, lime juice, chili, and garlic to a simmer. Add fish and shrimp. Simmer (do not boil) until fish is opaque and shrimp turn pink, about 2 minutes for the shrimp and 5 minutes for the fish. Remove from poaching liquid, place in a bowl, and cool in the refrigerator.

In the meantime, mix tomatoes, onion, jalapeño, lime juice, and cilantro together. Season to taste with hot sauce, salt, and pepper.

When the fish is cool, cut shrimp in half and cut fish into bite-sized pieces. Mix into tomato mixture. Chill for at least 1 hour, and up to 4 hours.

FAVORITE SHRIMP SCAMPI

Why not gather your favorite people this weekend and share this legendary recipe? They certainly will be slow to forget plump shrimp basted with a light garlic, herb, and lemon sauce. Serve accompanied by a light salad.

PREP TIME: 15 minutes. **COOKING TIME:** 8 minutes. Serves 4.

¾ cup organic olive oil

2 large cloves garlic, slivered

1 pound or more shrimp

2 large cloves garlic, minced

2 tbsp. fresh lemon juice

¼ cup fresh parsley, minced

1 tsp. salt or to taste

freshly ground pepper to taste

1 tbsp. dry sherry (optional)

In a large skillet, warm the olive oil over medium-low heat. Add the slivered garlic and cook gently, stirring occasionally. Add the shrimp and sprinkle with the minced garlic. Simmer for 1 to 2 minutes, then turn shrimp gently. Add the lemon juice, parsley, salt, pepper, and sherry. Increase the heat slightly and cook until shrimp are pink, about 2 minutes, stirring occasionally. Serve immediately.

SHRIMP IN RIESLING DIJON SAUCE

Recipe provided by Bonny Doon Vineyards. Serves 4-6.

PREP TIME: 15 minutes. **COOK TIME:** 3-4 minutes

3 tbsp. extra-virgin olive oil

3 tbsp. butter

4 cloves garlic, cut in half lengthwise

1 cup Dry Riesling (one brand is Pacific Rim)

2 tbsp. Dijon mustard

2 lbs. shrimp, shelled and deveined

Heat oil and butter in a large skillet until a haze forms. Add garlic and cook lightly. Remove garlic and discard. Add wine and bring to a boil. Lower heat and whisk in mustard. Add shrimp and cook until pink, 3 to 4 minutes.

QUINOA PAELLA

Quinoa comes from South America, and has been an important form of nourishment for more than 6,000 years. While it is technically not a grain, quinoa is grown and harvested for its seeds, and is used similarly to wheat and rice. It is a great source of protein, a complete source of balanced amino acids, and best of all it's easy to cook. It does, however, need to be thoroughly rinsed before cooking to remove a naturally occurring coating of bitter saponins. Once rinsed and cooked, quinoa is light and fluffy, and has a nutty flavor that tastes great in pilafs or salads, or as a hot breakfast cereal topped with yogurt, fresh fruit, and almonds. It's also easy to digest and gluten free. An ideal substitute for rice, bulgur, or couscous, quinoa is versatile and can be enjoyed in your favorite recipes.

PREP TIME: 15 minutes. **COOKING TIME:** 60 minutes. Serves 6.

1 onion, chopped	4 oz. black olives
2 minced garlic cloves or 1 tsp. minced garlic	1 cup organic peas
	3 cups organic chicken broth
¼ cup organic olive oil	Salt and red pepper, to taste
1½ cups organic quinoa, rinsed	2 sweet red peppers, sliced
⅛ tsp. saffron (or more to taste)	6 large, raw shrimp (or more)
2 cups cooked chicken, cut in 1- to 2-inch pieces	12 scrubbed clams, in shell
½ pound chorizo or other sausage (optional)	

Preheat oven to 350° F. In a medium-sized pan, sauté onion and garlic in half the olive oil. Add quinoa and saffron, and continue to sauté, stirring frequently. In a separate pan, sauté chicken and sausage in remaining olive oil until golden.

In a large casserole dish, mix together chicken, sausage, olives, peas, chicken broth, and quinoa mixture. Add salt and red pepper, if desired.

Cover and bake for 45 minutes or until quinoa has absorbed all liquid. Add sweet red peppers, shrimp, and clams. Cover and bake 10 additional minutes.

Other Quinoa Cooking Tips

Create a simple and delicious side dish for any meal by adding any of the following to cooked quinoa: sautéed onions; green pepper; mushrooms; toasted almonds, peanuts or other nuts; raisins or chopped dates; chopped parsley, cilantro, or other herbs.

POULTRY

GARLIC- & HERB-MARINATED CHICKEN BREASTS

MARINATE TIME: 2 hours or overnight. **COOKING TIME:** 15 minutes. Serves 4.

5 cloves garlic, minced	zest and juice of 1 lemon
1 tsp. basil	½ cup organic extra-virgin olive oil
1 tsp. thyme	1-gallon resealable plastic bag
1 tsp. oregano	6 boneless, skinless natural chicken
1 tsp. tarragon	breast halves
1 tsp. salt and pepper	grill brush and cooking oil

Mix together the first 7 ingredients in resealable plastic bag. Add chicken and marinate for 2 hours or overnight in refrigerator. Prepare a medium-hot fire in a grill. Brush grate with cooking oil. Place chicken on grill and sear 5 minutes per side or until it reaches 165° F.

ROASTED TURKEY BREAST
WITH GARAM MASALA RUB AND CITRUS SPICE GLAZE

Redolent with fragrant spices that are staples of Indian cuisine, this dish is not only delicious, it delivers AGE-reducing antioxidants with each bite.

PREP TIME: 20 minutes, plus 24 hours to marinate.

COOKING TIME: 2 hours. Serves 4 to 6.

GARAM MASALA

1 tablespoon each: ground coriander, ground cumin, ground black pepper, ground cayenne pepper, ground fennel, ground ginger, and ground cardamom.	1 teaspoon each: ground cloves and grated nutmeg

Mix spices together and store in a sealed container for up to 2 months.

TURKEY

1 (4- to 6-lb) all-natural turkey breast, thawed and rinsed	¼ to ½ c. garam masala
	1 large resealable plastic bag
2 tbsp. organic extra-virgin olive oil	

Rub turkey breast with olive oil. Rub spice mixture over the breast, including inside the breast cavity and underneath the skin. Place in resealable plastic bag and refrigerate overnight.

CITRUS SPICE GLAZE

1 cup organic orange juice	3 tbsp. honey
zest and juice of one orange	1 tbsp. garam masala
zest and juice of two limes	

Mix all ingredients in a small bowl and refrigerate until needed.

ROASTING THE TURKEY BREAST

Preheat oven to 350° F. Place turkey breast on rack in shallow roasting pan. Loosely tent foil around turkey breast and place in oven. Roast for 2 hours, or until the internal temperature reaches 170° F. Baste with glaze every half hour or so. Remove foil for last half hour of roasting (reserve foil). If pan gets dry, add an inch or so of water or chicken broth to the pan. Remove turkey breast from oven. Cover with foil. Let rest 20 minutes before carving.

EASY GRILLED CHICKEN BREASTS

This simple yet delicious recipe infuses lemon and olive oil to accent the naturally good flavor of fresh boneless, skinless chicken breast. Serve with baked squash, asparagus, or a crisp tossed salad.

PREP TIME: 1 hour. GRILLING TIME: 15 minutes. Serves 4.

4 boneless, skinless chicken breasts	1 tsp. salt
¼ cup organic olive oil	1 tsp. pepper
juice of 1 lemon	

Rinse chicken thoroughly with cool water. Mix olive oil, lemon, salt, and pepper thoroughly in large bowl. Immerse chicken in marinade. Then re-move one chicken breast at a time and put each in separate resealable bag. Marinate for 1 hour.

Heat grill or grill pan until it reaches medium heat. Remove chicken from plastic bags and cook each side for 6–8 minutes. Serve immediately alongside squash, asparagus, or a salad.

LIME-GRILLED CHICKEN WITH POMEGRANATE SALSA

TOTAL TIME: 30 minutes, plus 1 to 4 hours to marinate. Serves 4.

juice of 3 limes	1 large resealable plastic bag
1 clove garlic, minced	4 (6-oz.) all-natural boneless,
2 tbsp cilantro	skinless chicken breasts
¼ cup organic olive oil	canola oil

Mix lime juice, garlic, cilantro, and oil in a resealable plastic bag. Add chicken. Make sure chicken is evenly coated with marinade. Refrigerate for 1 to 4 hours. Heat grill or grill pan over medium heat. Brush lightly with canola oil. Cook chicken 7 minutes per side, or until the internal temperature reaches 165° F. Allow to rest 5 minutes before serving. Serve topped with Pomegranate Salsa.

POMEGRANATE SALSA

Makes about 1½ cups

3 tbsp. diced red onion	¼ cup pure pomegranate juice
1 clove garlic, minced	zest of one lime
1 tbsp. extra-virgin organic olive oil	½ cup chopped fresh cilantro
seeds from two pomegranates (about 1 cup)	salt and pepper to taste

Sauté onion and garlic in olive oil. Place in a bowl. Stir in pomegranate seeds, pomegranate juice, lime zest, and cilantro. Season to taste. Chill until needed.

MOROCCAN TURKEY STEW

A spice lover's paradise of a dish.

TOTAL TIME: 45 minutes. Serves 6.

1 tbsp. canola oil	1 tsp. turmeric
1 yellow onion, chopped	½ tsp. coriander
5 cloves garlic, minced	½ tsp ginger
2 carrots, peeled and sliced	½ tsp allspice
2 cups leftover (or fresh) roasted sweet potatoes, yams, or butternut squash	¼ tsp. freshly grated nutmeg
	2 tbsp. brown sugar
1 (15-oz.) can chickpeas	3 cups chicken broth
1 (28-oz.) can fire-roasted tomatoes	⅓ cup red wine (optional)
½ cup golden raisins, apricots, or dried cranberries	2 cups leftover turkey, cut into bite-sized pieces
1 tsp. salt	cooked couscous
1 tsp. cinnamon	½ cup slivered almonds
1 tsp. curry powder	¼ cup chopped mint and parsley
	1 cup plain yogurt

Heat oil in large soup pot. Add onion, garlic, and carrots. Cook 5 minutes, until soft. Add sweet potatoes, chick peas, tomatoes, raisins, spices, wine, and broth. Cover and simmer 20 minutes. Stir in turkey and cook 10 minutes longer. Adjust liquid and seasonings to taste.

Serve warm over couscous, topped with almonds, mint/parsley mixture, and a dollop of yogurt.

TOFU WITH EGGPLANT AND PEPPERS

Recipe provided by Bonny Doon Vineyards, courtesy of Wild Oats

As you have learned, it is not just meat and seafood flavors that can benefit from enjoyment with a glass of fine wine. This is a vegetarian recipe that is delightful with resveratrol-rich wines.

A scrumptious concoction of fresh vegetables and tofu, this traditional Vietnamese dish is excellent with earthy red wines such as our Domaine des Blagueurs Syrah Sirrah. Resveratrol, which occurs naturally in red wine, has powerful antiglycating properties.

PREP TIME: 45 minutes. **COOKING TIME:** 40 minutes. Serves 6.

1½ lbs. extra-firm tofu, drained and cut into 1-inch cubes	1 large eggplant, cut into 1-inch cubes
3 tbsp. peanut oil	1½ lbs. mushrooms
1 onion, chopped	2 summer squash, cut into 1-inch cubes
3 tbsp. soy sauce	
wafer (if necessary)	1 bunch of scallions, coarsely chopped (white and green parts)
3 large tomatoes, peeled and cut into eighths	1½ tbsp. tomato paste
3 large red peppers, chopped	6 fresh cilantro sprigs, for garnish
1 small jalapeño or other hot pepper, seeded and minced	

Place tofu cubes into a steamer and allow to steam for 20 to 30 minutes while chopping vegetables.

Meanwhile, heat oil in a wok or large skillet until hot. Transfer tofu to pan and sauté until golden on all sides, then remove from pan and set aside.

In same pan, sauté onion for one minute. Add soy sauce and one tablespoon water if necessary. Add tomatoes, red peppers, hot pepper, eggplant, mushrooms, squash, scallions, and tomato paste and reduce heat. Simmer for about 10 minutes, or until vegetables are soft. Add tofu and continue cooking until tofu is heated through.

Serve on platter, garnished with cilantro.

SQUARE MEALS IN A ROUND BOWL

These savory salads and soups make a complete meal or hearty first course.

GREEK SALMON SALAD

Savor the flamboyant flavors of the Greek isles with this simply super salmon salad. It's nutritional levels reach Olympic proportions, rejuvenating and refueling your body.

PREP TIME: 15 minutes. Serves 4.

3 tbsp. organic olive oil	1 cup red pepper, diced
2 tbsp. red wine vinegar or fresh lemon juice	⅛ cup purple onion, finely diced
1 tbsp. organic Dijon mustard	1 cucumber, peeled, seeded, and diced
2 tsp. oregano	8 kalamata olives, pitted and diced
1 tsp. dill	¼ cup feta cheese, crumbled
salt and freshly ground pepper to taste	2 cups romaine lettuces, torn into bite-sized pieces
1 can (15.5-oz) wild salmon, drained	

In large bowl, whisk together the olive oil, vinegar or lemon juice, mustard, oregano, dill, salt, and pepper. Gently fold in the salmon, red pepper, onion, cucumber, olives, and feta. Serve on top of lettuce.

CELERY ROOT SALAD
WITH SMOKED SALMON AND CREAMY DIJON DRESSING

HOMEMADE MAYONNAISE

Makes 1 cup

2 large organic, free-range, cage-free, omega-3 egg yolks	$\frac{1}{4}$ tsp. sea salt
	dash of white pepper
3 tbsp. lemon juice, freshly squeezed	1 cup olive oil

Place yolks, lemon juice, salt, and pepper in a mixing bowl. Whisk in oil, a couple of drops at a time, to create an emulsion. After about a third of the oil is incorporated, add the rest in a steady stream, while whisking. Place in a glass jar, cover, and refrigerate until needed.

CREAMY DIJON DRESSING

1 cup homemade mayonnaise	1 anchovy, finely chopped
2 tsp. organic Dijon mustard	1 tsp. white wine vinegar
1 tbsp. capers, chopped	2 tbsp. tarragon, chopped (reserve 2 tsp. for garnish)
2 cornichons, finely chopped	
juice of one lemon	Sea salt and pepper to taste

Combine mayonnaise with mustard, capers, cornichons, lemon juice, anchovy, vinegar, and tarragon. Mix thoroughly. Season with salt and pepper.

SALAD

Serves 2.

1 organic celery root, peeled and thinly sliced	2 oz. hot smoked salmon, sliced

Toss celery root with enough Dijon dressing to evenly coat. Portion between two plates and garnish with slices of smoked salmon. Sprinkle with fresh tarragon.

FIVE-BEAN SALAD

TOTAL TIME: 20 minutes. Serves 12 to 15.

2 cups organic shelled edamame (salted, boiled green soybeans)

1 (16-oz.) bag organic green beans

1 (15-oz.) can organic dark red kidney beans, drained and rinsed

1 (15-oz.) can organic chickpeas, drained and rinsed

1 (15-oz.) can organic black beans, drained and rinsed

1 cup diced organic red onion

1 red, yellow, or orange pepper, diced

¼ cup organic Italian flat leaf parsley, chopped

8 leaves basil, chopped

1 (12-oz.) jar organic balsamic vinaigrette dressing

sea salt and black pepper to taste

1 (4-oz.) log of Herbes de Provence goat cheese, crumbled (or another brand)

Bring a large pot of salted water to a boil. Add the edamame and cook for 2 minutes. Thirty seconds before they are done, add the green beans. Drain and rinse under icy cold water. Place in a large salad bowl. Add the kidney beans, chickpeas, black beans, onion, peppers, parsley, and basil. Toss to distribute evenly. Add enough dressing to coat evenly. Add salt and pepper to taste. Garnish with crumbled goat cheese. Best served chilled.

HEIRLOOM TOMATO AND FRESH MOZZARELLA STACK WITH BALSAMIC VINAIGRETTE

PREP TIME: 15 minutes. Serves 4.

1 tbsp. 12-Star balsamic vinegar (or another brand)

4 tbsp. organic extra-virgin olive oil

2 tbsp. fresh basil, chopped

1 tsp. oregano

1 clove garlic, minced or pressed

4 to 6 large heirloom, organic, or on-the-vine tomatoes

8 oz. fresh mozzarella

salt and freshly cracked pepper to taste

2 tbsp. fresh basil, chopped

Mix first five ingredients together and set aside. Slice tomatoes into ½-inch slices. Slice mozzarella into 8 slices. Alternately layer tomatoes and mozzarella. Drizzle each salad with vinaigrette and season with salt and pepper. Garnish with fresh basil.

SOUTHWEST QUINOA CHOPPED SALAD WITH CHICKEN AND CREAMY SALSA DRESSING

PREP TIME: 25 minutes. Serves 6.

1 cup organic quinoa	1 cup organic black beans, rinsed
1 tsp. sea salt	½ organic red or orange bell pepper, diced
1 cup medium salsa	
¼ cup organic plain yogurt	1 avocado, chopped
3 tbsp. chopped cilantro	1 large ripe organic tomato, chopped
2 tsp. extra-virgin olive oil	
juice and zest of one organic lime	1 large head organic romaine, chopped
sea salt to taste	
2 cups rotisserie chicken, chopped into bite-sized pieces	chopped lime wedges and cilantro for garnish

Bring 1½ cups of cold water to a boil. Place quinoa in a fine-mesh strainer and rinse thoroughly under cold water. Place quinoa and salt in boiling water. Bring back to a boil. Cover and reduce heat to a simmer. Cook for about 15 minutes. Turn off the heat and let sit covered for about 5 minutes. Drain quinoa in fine-mesh strainer and set aside to cool.

Place salsa, yogurt, cilantro, olive oil, lime juice, and zest in a blender. Pulse until smooth. Season with salt. Place in refrigerator to chill.

Toss cooled quinoa with chicken, beans, pepper, avocado, and tomato. Add just enough dressing to coat evenly.

Divide romaine on six plates and top with quinoa salad mixture.

Garnish with wedges of fresh lime and cilantro.

ASIAN CRUNCH SALAD WITH GRILLED TURKEY TENDERLOIN

This salad is a delicious meal made with a number of superfoods. The almonds are high in protein, fiber, calcium, magnesium, potassium, vitamin E, and other antioxidants and phytochemicals. They are also an excellent source of healthy fats. The turkey is an excellent source of lean protein, and the cabbage is a great source of dietary fiber and complex carbohydrates. Cabbage also instructs our genes to increase production of the enzyme that detoxifies the body—this could help accelerate the removal of dietary AGEs.

PREP TIME: 20 minutes. Serves 1.

TURKEY SALAD

4 oz. natural turkey tenderloin

2 tbsp. Wild Oats Organic Asian sesame marinade (or other brand)

½ tsp. olive oil

ASIAN-STYLE GINGER DRESSING

1½ tbsp. olive oil

1 tbsp. rice wine vinegar

1 tsp. low-sodium soy sauce

1 tsp. fresh organic ginger, grated

SALAD

2 tbsp. organic green onions, diced

½ tsp. sesame seeds, toasted

½ cup organic napa cabbage, thinly sliced

1 small organic carrot, shredded

1 tbsp. organic slivered almonds, toasted

Marinate turkey in Asian marinade for 20 minutes.

Heat grill pan over medium heat. Add ½ tsp. oil. Place turkey in pan. Sear each side for 5 to 6 minutes, or until the internal temperature reaches 165° F. Let turkey rest 5 minutes before slicing.

In a bowl, whisk together dressing ingredients. Toss salad vegetables in dressing and top with turkey.

SALMON AND SOBA NOODLE BOWL
IN A SPICY GINGER MISO BROTH

If you miss the delicious taste of noodles, take heart. Soba noodles are made from buckwheat, a gluten-free and wheat-free grain. Soba noodles are a slow-releasing carbohydrate.

TOTAL TIME: 30 minutes. Serves 4.

6 cups organic chicken or vegetable broth

8 oz. soba noodles

1 tbsp. minced ginger

2 garlic cloves, minced

1 tbsp. low-sodium soy sauce

1 tbsp. fish sauce

1 Thai chili, thinly sliced

4 baby bok choy, quartered

¼ cup shredded organic carrots

1 lb. wild salmon fillet, cut into 1-inch cubes

1 cup bean sprouts

2 tbsp. yellow or white miso

sesame oil for garnish

2 tsp. sesame seeds for garnish

4 tbsp. chopped cilantro for garnish

Bring broth to a boil in a large saucepan. Add soba noodles and cook 8 minutes. Remove noodles from stock using a mesh ladle, reserving stock, rinse under cold water, and set noodles aside.

Add ginger, garlic, soy sauce, fish sauce, chili, bok choy, and carrots to the broth. Simmer for 6 minutes, until bok choy is soft. Add salmon, sprouts, and miso. Cook 2 to 3 minutes, until salmon is just cooked (do not let the broth boil).

Divide noodles between 4 bowls and top with salmon, vegetables, and broth.

Garnish with a drizzle of sesame oil, sesame seeds, and cilantro.

30-MINUTE TOMATO BISQUE

Say good-bye to winter's chill with steaming bowls of creamy tomato bisque, guaranteed to warm you from your taste buds to your toes. Made with organic tomatoes, preserved at peak ripeness, this soup brings a little sunshine to a dreary winter day. And it's ready in 30 minutes!

PREP TIME: 10 minutes. **COOKING TIME:** 20 minutes. Serves 4 to 6.

3 tbsp. extra-virgin olive oil	1 tbsp. basil
½ tsp. red pepper flakes	1 (28-oz.) can diced tomatoes
1 medium organic yellow onion, diced	1 (28-oz.) can crushed tomatoes with basil
6 cloves garlic, minced	3 tbsp. tomato paste
3 bay leaves	½ cup yogurt
2 tsp. thyme	sea salt and black pepper to taste

Heat oil in a large saucepan over medium heat. Add red pepper flakes. Cook for about 30 seconds to infuse the oil with the spice. Add onion and garlic. Cook for about 5 minutes, or until very soft. Add bay leaves, thyme, and basil. Stir. Add tomatoes and tomato paste. Stir. Cover and simmer for 10 minutes. Remove bay leaves. Puree about half the soup in a blender, or use a handheld blender and blend to a chunky puree. Stir in yogurt. Season with salt and pepper. Taste and adjust seasonings. Ladle into bowls and serve.

CIOPPINI VERSION 1

Originally created by Italian-American fishermen in San Francisco to use up odds and ends of the catch of the day, cioppino is a rich tomato-based stew chock-full of seafood and scented with basil, oregano, and marjoram. Add a crisp salad and robust merlot or fruity Chianti for a truly memorable feast to share with family and friends.

You can make the broth ahead of time and freeze it until you're ready to make the stew. Just thaw, bring to a boil, and add the fish according to the recipe. This is one of my favorite meals and one that has many variations. I have included two versions for your dining pleasure.

PREP TIME: 15 minutes. **COOKING TIME:** 45 minutes. Serves 6 to 8.

---

1 tbsp. extra-virgin olive oil

red pepper flakes to taste

6 cloves garlic, minced

1 small bulb fennel, diced (about ½ cup)

1 small onion, diced

1 (28-oz.) can fire-roasted tomatoes, diced (one brand is Muir Glen)

1 (14-oz.) can organic tomato puree

2 tbsp. organic tomato paste

1 cup red wine

2 tsp. basil

2 tsp. oregano

1 tsp. marjoram

2 tbsp. organic unsalted butter or extra-virgin olive oil

3 tbsp. flat-leaf Italian parsley, chopped

sea salt and pepper to taste

1 lb. crab legs

1 large lobster tail meat, cut into 1-inch chunks

1 lb. sea bass, cut into 1-inch chunks

1 lb. mussels, debearded and with one half of the shell removed and discarded

12–14 clams, one half of the shell removed and discarded

½ lb. extra-large shrimp, peeled and thawed

½ lb. scallops

parsley, for garnish

In a large soup pot, heat olive oil over medium heat. Add red pepper flakes, garlic, fennel, and onion. Cook for about 10 minutes, until onion is very soft.

Add diced tomatoes, tomato puree, and tomato paste. Stir in wine, basil, oregano, and marjoram. Cover and simmer for 20 to 30 minutes. Stir in butter or olive oil and seasonings and adjust to taste. Add crab, lobster, and sea bass. Bring to a boil. Cover and cook on low heat for 8 minutes.

Add mussels, clams, shrimp, and scallops. Cover and cook for 2 minutes. Garnish with parsley.

Set the soup pot on the table with a big ladle and appropriate seafood tools. Enjoy!

CIOPPINO VERSION 2

PREP TIME: 10 minutes. **COOKING TIME:** 45 minutes. Serves 12 to 14.

¾ cup organic extra-virgin olive oil

2 organic onions, chopped

2 cloves garlic, minced

1 bunch fresh parsley, chopped

2 (14.5-ounce) cans stewed tomatoes

2 (14.5-ounce) cans chicken broth

2 bay leaves

1 tbsp. dried basil

½ tsp. dried thyme

½ tsp. dried oregano

1 cup water

1½ cups white wine

1½ pounds large shrimp, peeled and deveined

1½ pounds bay scallops

18 small clams

18 mussels, cleaned and debearded

1½ cups crabmeat

1½ pounds cod fillets, cubed (optional)

Over medium-low heat, heat olive oil in a large pot, then add onions, garlic, and parsley. Cook slowly, stirring occasionally until onions are soft.

Add tomatoes to the pot (break them into chunks as you add them). Add chicken broth, bay leaves, basil, thyme, oregano, water, and wine. Mix well. Cover and simmer 30 minutes.

Stir in the shrimp, scallops, clams, mussels, and crabmeat. Stir in fish, if desired. Bring to boil. Lower heat, cover, and simmer 5 to 7 minutes until clams open. Ladle soup into bowls.

CURRIED BUTTERNUT SQUASH AND COCONUT BISQUE

PREP TIME: 20 minutes. **COOKING TIME:** 25 minutes. Serves 6.

½ cup toasted coconut for garnish

2 tbsp. organic unsalted butter

1 medium organic yellow onion, diced

2 cloves garlic, minced

2 tbsp. curry powder

1 tsp. cinnamon

½ tsp. allspice

4 cups organic butternut squash, peeled and cubed

2½ cups organic vegetable or chicken broth

1 cup organic coconut milk

zest of one lime

sea salt and pepper

½ cup chopped cilantro, for garnish

Heat skillet over medium-high heat. Add coconut to pan. Toast lightly. Remove from pan and set aside.

Melt butter in large saucepan over medium heat. Add onion and garlic. Cook until tender, stirring occasionally (about 10 minutes). Stir in curry powder and allspice. Cook for about one minute. Add butternut squash and chicken broth. Bring to a boil, then reduce heat to medium-low. Cover and simmer for 25 minutes, or until squash is tender, stirring occasionally.

Working in batches, carefully puree soup in blender until smooth.

Return soup to the pot and stir in coconut milk and lime zest. Add salt and pepper to taste.

Garnish with coconut and cilantro.

SOUTHERN INDIA CHICKEN CURRY

PREP TIME: 15 minutes. **COOKING TIME:** 40 minutes. Serves 4 to 6.

2 tbsp. canola oil

1 medium yellow onion, diced

3 tbsp. ginger, peeled and minced

2 cloves garlic, minced

2 lbs. boneless, skinless chicken breast

½ red pepper, thinly sliced

3 cups coconut milk

2 cups organic chicken broth

1 cup cooked chickpeas

2 bay leaves

2 tbsp. turmeric

2 tbsp. curry powder

½ tsp. cinnamon

2 tbsp. lime juice

hot chili sauce to taste

½ cup cilantro, chopped

In a large pot lightly sauté onion, ginger, and garlic in oil for 4 minutes. Cut chicken into 2-inch chunks. Add chicken and pepper to pot. Cook for 2 minutes. Add coconut milk, broth, chickpeas, bay leaves, turmeric, curry powder, cinnamon, lime juice, and chili sauce. Simmer for 30 minutes. Stir in cilantro.

FIERY BUFFALO CHILI

This hearty meal can be made with all-natural ground buffalo, or organic free-range ground turkey or chicken. For a vegetarian dish, just omit the meat.

PREP TIME: 1.5 hours. **COOKING TIME:** 1 hour. Serves 6.

2 tbsp. olive oil

2 medium onions, diced (about
  2 cups)

1 medium zucchini, diced (about
  ½ cup)

1 medium yellow squash, diced (about
  ½ cup)

2 cloves garlic, minced

2 lbs. natural ground buffalo

2 (28-ounce) cans of diced natural
  tomatoes

1 (6-ounce) can natural tomato paste

2 (15-ounce) cans organic kidney
  beans

4 tbsp. chili powder

1 tbsp. cumin

1 tsp. cayenne (optional)

2 tsp. sea salt

water or beer (if necessary)

1 (8-ounce) package raw milk cheddar
  cheese, shredded

1 (8-ounce) cup yogurt

1 bunch fresh cilantro, chopped

Heat a large soup pot over medium heat. Add oil, onion, zucchini, squash, and garlic. Sauté for 5 minutes, or until soft. Add buffalo. Cook and stir until brown. Add diced tomatoes, tomato paste, beans, chili powder, cumin, cayenne, and salt. If chili is too thick, add water or beer to achieve desired consistency. Simmer for at least 1 hour.

Ladle into bowls and serve piping hot.

Garnish with cheddar cheese, yogurt, and chopped cilantro.

GREEK SALAD WITH SOUVLAKI

Re-create the zesty flavors of Greek cuisine with this world-class dish. As always, you can substitute tofu for any meat.

PREP TIME: 25 minutes, plus 2 hours to marinate. **COOKING TIME:** 10 minutes.
Serves 6.

SOUVLAKI

2 lemons, juiced	2 cloves garlic, minced
1 tbsp. lemon zest	salt and pepper
½ cup olive oil	2 lbs. natural pork tenderloin
2 tsp. oregano, minced	12 wooden skewers, soaked in water

Mix together the first six ingredients in a bowl. Cut pork into 2-inch cubes and add to marinade. Cover and refrigerate for 2 hours.

Thread pork onto skewers. Gently grill skewers on a grill pan, 4 to 6 minutes on each side.

VINAIGRETTE

4 tbsp. olive oil	1 clove garlic, minced
4 tbsp. red wine vinegar	1 tsp. mint, minced
2 tsp. oregano, minced	salt and pepper to taste

Whisk all the ingredients together.

SALAD

1 head organic romaine, rinsed and torn into bite-sized pieces	15 grape tomatoes, halved
½ red onion, thinly sliced	15 kalamata olives, pitted and halved
2 cucumbers, peeled, halved, seeded, and sliced	1 cup feta cheese, crumbled

Toss first five ingredients together. Add vinaigrette. Plate and top with feta and skewers.

CYPRESS SALAD

It's important to buy organic produce—such as salad greens—as salad greens can have high levels of pesticides. Always wash all of your fruits and veggies before use.

PREP TIME: 15 minutes. **COOKING TIME:** 5 minutes. Serves 4.

BRUSCHETTA TOPPING

1½ lbs ripe juicy tomatoes

1 garlic clove, minced

1–2 tbsp. capers, rinsed

¼ cup loosely packed fresh oregano or fresh basil

sea salt and freshly ground pepper to taste

⅓ cup extra-virgin olive oil

6 cups organic spring salad mix

1 cup prepared Bruschetta Topping

⅓ to ½ cup Fire-Roasted Tomato Dressing (see recipe p. 314)

1 (5-oz.) natural chicken breast, baked and sliced

2 slices natural deli ham, sliced thick and chopped

2 slices natural turkey, sliced thick and chopped

2 strips natural uncured nitrate-free turkey bacon, cooked and chopped

1 slice natural Swiss cheese, sliced and chopped

¼ cup feta cheese, crumbled

Balsamic Tomato Glaze (see recipe p. 314)

Bring medium saucepan of water to a boil. Cut across tomatoes at the root end and drop them into the boiling water. Cook until skin of tomatoes begins to split, 1 to 2 minutes. Transfer tomatoes to bowl of iced water. Peel and seed tomatoes, then roughly chop. Place in strainer over bowl for 20 to 30 minutes. Put tomatoes, garlic, capers, and oregano or basil in bowl. Season with salt and pepper. Add oil and mix.

In a large mixing bowl, toss together spring salad mix and bruschetta topping with just enough Fire-Roasted Tomato Dressing to lightly coat the greens. Divide greens between four plates and top each salad with equal amounts of chicken, ham, turkey, bacon, Swiss cheese, and feta. Drizzle with Balsamic Tomato Glaze, grab a fork, and enjoy!

FIRE-ROASTED TOMATO DRESSING

PREP TIME: 5 minutes. **COOKING TIME:** 5 minutes. Makes about 1 cup.

½ cup fire-roasted canned diced tomatoes, drained

6 fresh basil leaves

4 tbsp. organic brown rice vinegar or balsamic vinegar

1 tsp. Cajun seasoning blend

½ clove garlic

2 tbsp. organic green onions, finely chopped

pinch of agave nectar to taste

⅓ cup organic extra-virgin olive oil

4 tbsp. organic canola mayonnaise

sea salt and freshly cracked pepper to taste

Place tomatoes, basil, vinegar, Cajun seasoning, garlic, onions, and agave nectar in a blender or food processor. Pulse until pureed. While blender or food processor is running, slowly add olive oil until mixture thickens. Add mayonnaise and pulse until just mixed and creamy. Add salt and pepper. Adjust seasonings to taste. Store in a glass, airtight container for up to one week in the refrigerator.

Tip: Add 3 or 4 oil-packed sun-dried tomatoes for even richer tomato flavor.

BALSAMIC TOMATO GLAZE

PREP TIME: 5 minutes. **COOKING TIME:** 4 minutes. Makes ½ cup.

⅓ cup organic tomato paste

2 tbsp. balsamic vinegar

½ clove garlic, minced

agave nectar to taste

2 tsp. lime juice

Whisk together all ingredients in a saucepan over medium heat. Bring to a boil for 3 minutes, stirring constantly. Remove from heat and put into storage container. Place container into an ice bath or refrigerator to cool. Once the glaze is cool, place into a squeeze bottle for better presentation on salad. Keep refrigerated.

EARTH AND SEA SALAD

Sea vegetables are rich in minerals and trace elements, including calcium, magnesium, iron, potassium, iodine, manganese, and chromium, at levels much greater than those found in land vegetables. They contain the B-vitamins folate, riboflavin, and pantothenic acid, and like flax and pumpkin seeds, they are rich in lignans, phytochemicals with cancer-protective properties. Sea veggies also provide vitamins, fiber, enzymes, and high-quality protein. They have a delicate flavor.

PREP TIME: 90 minutes. Serves 4.

2 cups dried arame

1 cup dried hijiki

½ cup julienned red pepper

½ cup chopped scallions

½ cup raw organic carrots, jullienned

½ cup cucumbers, peeled, seeded, and sliced

½ pound organic tofu

1 tbsp. organic sesame seeds

JAPANESE DRESSING

½ cup low-sodium soy sauce

½ cup rice vinegar

½ cup mirin

½ cup sesame oil

2 tbsp. fresh grated ginger

Soak the arame and hijiki for 30 minutes. Squeeze out water and pick out any foreign matter. Simmer in boiling water for 30 minutes or until tender. Drain and set aside to cool.

Meanwhile, mix Japanese dressing and set aside. Chop vegetables.

Cut tofu into strips.

Combine seaweed with vegetables, tofu, sesame seeds, and Japanese dressing. Let rest 30 minutes and toss before serving.

CHILLED SOBA NOODLE SALAD
WITH GREEN CURRY AND JAPANESE TOFU

This salad is delicious hot or cold, and is great with shrimp or chicken as well as tofu. Red curry paste also works in place of the green. Soba noodles are made from buckwheat, and are a good source of protein, potassium, and iron—and they are low glycemic, which means they will not promote AGE formation. Soba noodles are tasty in chilled salads, steamy soups, and spicy stir-fries. They are a great low-glycemic alternative to rice noodles and traditional pasta.

TOTAL TIME: 25 minutes. Serves 4.

8 oz. soba noodles

½ cup sugar snap peas or pea pods,
    thinly sliced

½ red pepper, thinly sliced

⅓ cup bean sprouts

½ lb. Japanese tofu salad or your
    favorite marinated and baked tofu,
    chopped into bite-sized pieces

2 tsp. canola oil

1 stalk lemongrass, roughly chopped

2 cloves garlic, minced

1 tbsp. ginger, minced

2 tbsp. green curry paste (to taste)

16 oz. organic coconut milk

¼ cup chopped cilantro

Cook soba noodles according to package instructions. When done, drain and run under very cold water to chill. Place in a bowl.

Place pea pods, red pepper, bean sprouts, and tofu on top of noodles.

Heat oil in a large saucepan. Add lemongrass, garlic, and ginger. Cook for 1 minute. Add curry paste. Cook for 1 minute. Stir in coconut milk and simmer for about 5 minutes.

Strain through a fine-mesh strainer. Discard ginger, garlic, and lemongrass.

Pour hot curry over noodles and vegetables. Stir together and chill for at least an hour.

Serve cold, topped with cilantro.

SAVORY SIDES

A study at Georgetown University that was published in the *British Journal of Cancer* found that indole-3-carbinol, a chemical in vegetables such as cabbage, broccoli sprouts, Brussels sprouts, cauliflower, bok choy, and kale, actually boosts DNA repair in cells and may stop them from becoming cancerous. DNA is the material inside the nucleus of the cells that contains our genetic information. If one is genetically predisposed to cancer, it might be possible to boost the repair mechanism in one's DNA and thus prevent cancer—more good reasons to love your vegetables.

BRUSSELS SPROUTS WITH THREE-CITRUS BUTTER

TOTAL TIME: 15 minutes. Serves 8.

3 lbs. Brussels sprouts, trimmed and sliced in half

½ stick unsalted butter or ¼ stick butter and ¼ cup olive oil

2 tsp. organic lemon zest

2 tsp. organic orange zest

2 tsp. organic tangerine zest

salt and pepper to taste

Cook Brussels sprouts in a large saucepan of salted boiling water for about 5 to 6 minutes. Drain and place on a platter. Melt butter in a saucepan. Stir in citrus zest. Pour over Brussels sprouts. Season with salt and pepper. Serve immediately.

SESAME GINGER KALE

TOTAL TIME: 15 minutes. Serves 4 to 5.

1 tbsp. organic extra-virgin olive oil

3 cloves minced garlic

3 tbsp. low-sodium soy sauce or tamari

1 tbsp. minced ginger

2 tsp. sesame oil

1 tsp. red pepper flakes or Asian-style hot sauce

1½ lbs. kale, stemmed, rinsed, and chopped

⅓ cup vegetable broth, chicken broth, or water

2 tbsp. lightly toasted sesame seeds

Heat oil in a large wok or sauté pan over medium-high heat. Stir in garlic, soy sauce, ginger, sesame oil, and red pepper flakes. Add kale, tossing to coat lightly. Add vegetable broth, cover, and cook for 5 minutes or until kale is tender. Stir in sesame seeds, remove from wok, and enjoy immediately.

ASPARAGUS AND SPRING PEA TOSS

PREP TIME: 10 minutes. **COOKING TIME:** 6 minutes. Serves 6.

1 tbsp. sea salt

2 lbs. organic asparagus

1 cup fresh organic peas, shelled

4 tbsp. organic unsalted butter

⅓ cup parmigiano-Reggiano cheese, grated

2 tsp. lemon zest

2 tbsp. fresh mint, minced

sea salt and freshly ground black pepper

Fill a large saucepan half full of water. Add salt and bring to a boil. Clean asparagus and break off woody ends. Cut into 1½-inch pieces. Reduce heat to a simmer. Add asparagus and simmer for 2 minutes. Add peas and cook 30 seconds longer. Drain and place in a bowl. Add butter, cheese, lemon, and mint. Toss to coat evenly. Season with salt and pepper.

SWISS CHARD WITH WALNUTS, LEMON, AND GOAT CHEESE

TOTAL TIME: 15 minutes. Serves 4.

1 tbsp. organic olive oil

2 cloves garlic, minced

1 lb. chard, cleaned, trimmed, chopped, with stems separated from leaves

⅓ cup organic chicken or vegetable broth

4 tbsp. chopped walnuts

zest of one lemon

1 tbsp. 12 Star balsamic vinegar

Salt and pepper to taste

2 oz. goat cheese, crumbled

Heat oil in a large skillet over medium heat. Add garlic and chard stems. Add broth. Cover and steam 3 minutes. Add chard leaves, and cook 2 minutes, until wilted. Stir in walnuts, lemon zest, and balsamic vinegar. Season with salt and pepper. Remove from heat and top with goat cheese.

SAUTÉED SPINACH WITH GARLIC AND LEMON

Spinach has long been one of my favorite vegetables. But I'm not talking about the overcooked mush served at cafeteria steam tables, which also results from cooking frozen spinach. Ideally, you should choose fresh spinach and serve it lightly sautéed to preserve its nutrients and appealing deep-green color.

But there is much more to spinach than good taste. Calorie for calorie, spinach and other dark-green leafy vegetables provide more preventive-health nutrients and anti-aging antioxidants than most other foods. Spinach is one of the vegetables that has the highest amount of chlorophyll, a fat-soluble substance that stimulates hemoglobin and red blood cell production.

Spinach is also extraordinarily rich in a variety of powerfully antioxidant, anti-inflammatory phytonutrients, including flavonoids like quercetin and carotenoids such as beta-carotene and lutein. Spinach is also excellent for sharpening the mind. Researchers at Tufts University report that men who consumed foods high in folate (such as spinach) for three years displayed sharper cognitive skills at the end of the study period.

PREP TIME: 15 minutes. **COOKING TIME:** 4 minutes. Serves 8.

2 tbsp. olive oil	sea salt and black pepper
4 cloves minced garlic	fresh lemon wedges
2 lbs. baby spinach leaves, coarse stems discarded, washed well and drained in a colander	

Heat a large skillet over medium heat. Add the oil and sauté garlic 1 minute, until soft. Add spinach and cook 2 to 3 minutes, turning with tongs until bright green and just wilted. Season with salt and pepper and freshly squeezed lemon juice. Serve immediately.

SPINACH ARTICHOKE DIP

TOTAL TIME: 1 hour. Serves 8.

1 (14-oz.) can artichoke hearts or
  bottoms, drained and rinsed

1 (10-oz.) package frozen chopped
  spinach, thawed

1 roasted red pepper, chopped

½ cup parmigiano-Reggiano

½ cup low-fat cheddar or Monterrey
  Jack cheese

⅓ cup light canola mayonnaise

4 cloves garlic, minced

Preheat oven to 350° F. Chop artichoke parts into small pieces and place in mixing bowl. Place spinach in a clean dish towel and wring over the kitchen sink to remove excess water. Place spinach in bowl. Add red pepper, cheeses, mayonnaise, and garlic. Mix until just combined. Place in baking dish and cover with lid or foil. Bake 30 minutes, until bubbling. Remove foil and bake 10 minutes longer, until golden. Serve with fresh crudités.

BARLEY AND SPINACH PILAF

PREP TIME: 10 minutes. **COOKING TIME:** 60 minutes. Serves 6 to 8.

1½ tbsp. organic unsalted butter

1½ tbsp olive oil

1 cup organic barley

½ cup red onion, finely chopped

1 clove garlic, minced

6 oz. organic mushrooms, chopped

3 cups organic vegetable broth

8 oz. organic baby spinach

salt and pepper to taste

¼ cup pecans, chopped

Melt butter and olive oil in a large saucepan. Stir in barley and cook for 1 minute. Add onion, garlic, and mushrooms. Cook for about 5 minutes. Add broth and bring to a boil. Cover, reduce heat to medium-low, and simmer 45 to 55 minutes or until liquid is absorbed and barley is tender. Or place in covered casserole and bake at 350° F for 40 minutes. Stir in spinach 4 minutes before barley is done. Add salt and pepper to taste. Top with pecans and serve.

QUINOA PILAF WITH BABY SPINACH, PINE NUTS, AND BASIL

PREP TIME: 10 minutes. **COOKING TIME:** 30 minutes. Serves 6.

2 tbsp. olive oil	2 cups quinoa, rinsed 3 times
1 medium onion, finely chopped	4 cups chicken or vegetable broth
2 cloves garlic, minced	¼ cup pine nuts
½ red bell pepper, finely diced	3 tbsp. fresh basil, chopped
1 (10-oz.) bag organic baby spinach	sea salt and ground black pepper

Heat oil in a large skillet over medium heat. Add onion, garlic, and red pepper. Cook for 3 to 5 minutes, or until the peppers are soft. Add spinach and cook until it wilts. Add quinoa and broth. Bring to a boil over high heat. Reduce heat to a simmer, cover, and cook for 20 minutes, or until the quinoa is tender and the water is absorbed. Stir in pine nuts and basil. Season with salt and pepper. Fluff quinoa with a fork and serve.

BREAKFAST AND BRUNCH

Eggs can be a terrific source of protein and omega-3 essential fatty acids. The key is to make sure you purchase eggs from cage-free chickens that are fed flax meal. Not only are they much more nutritious, they taste wonderful.

A hard-boiled egg and an apple make a great snack—healthy carbs and fiber from the apple (remember that apples have excellent blood sugar–stabilizing abilities) and protein and healthy fat from the egg.

PERFECT HARD-BOILED EGGS

COOKING TIME: 20 minutes. Makes one dozen hard-boiled eggs.

Gently place a dozen eggs in a saucepan and cover with cold water. Bring to a boil and immediately remove from heat. Cover and let eggs stand for 10 to 12 minutes. Place eggs in a colander under ice-cold running water for a minute or two. Use immediately or place back in carton and refrigerate until ready to use.

ASPARAGUS AND AGED GOUDA MINI FRITTATAS

TOTAL TIME: 40 minutes. Makes 12.

cooking spray

¼ lb. asparagus, ends trimmed

2 tsp. olive oil

¼ cup diced onion

2 cloves garlic, minced

1 tsp. dried thyme

salt and black pepper to taste

5 large egg whites

3 large eggs

⅓ cup organic milk

1 tsp. baking powder

¾ cup shredded aged Gouda

paprika

Preheat oven to 375° F. Spray regular muffin pan with cooking spray. Slice asparagus in half lengthwise and chop into ½-inch pieces. Fill a sauté pan with two inches of water. Bring to a boil. Add asparagus and cook 3 minutes, until bright green and tender. Drain and place in a bowl of ice water.

Heat oil in sauté pan. Add onion and garlic. Cook 3 minutes, until soft. Stir in asparagus, thyme, salt, and pepper.

In a separate bowl, whisk eggs with milk and baking powder. Stir in vegetables and cheese.

Divide egg mixture evenly between muffin cups. Sprinkle with paprika. Bake 20 to 25 minutes, until firm to the touch.

EASY EGG SCRAMBLE

PREP TIME: 10 minutes. **COOKING TIME:** 5 minutes. Serves 4.

When you're trying to get out the door in the morning, try this recipe next time instead of skipping breakfast. It's easy and delicious.

4 cage-free eggs

¼ cup organic milk

1 tbsp. olive oil

3 medium-sized shallots, chopped

1 clove garlic, diced

½ cup Parmesan cheese, grated

salt and pepper to taste

Whip eggs and milk in large bowl. In large skillet heat olive oil over medium heat and sauté shallots until translucent, stirring frequently. Add chopped garlic and continue to sauté until fragrant.

Pour eggs into skillet and cover with lid for 30 seconds. Remove lid and with large spoon stir egg mixture, making sure to scrape mixture off bottom of pan. Continue to cover and mix until scrambled to desired consistency. Serve hot with grated Parmesan cheese and salt and pepper to taste.

VEGGIE AND CHEESE OMELET

PREP TIME: 15 minutes. **COOKING TIME:** 4 minutes. Serves 2.

2 large cage-free eggs	2 tbsp. organic red pepper, chopped
1 egg white or 3 egg whites, beaten	2 tbsp. organic broccoli, chopped
1 tsp. tarragon	2 tbsp. organic zucchini, chopped
salt and pepper to taste	2 tbsp. organic mushrooms, chopped
nonstick cooking spray	1 oz. low-fat cheddar cheese

Mix eggs with tarragon, salt, and pepper; set aside. Lightly spray pan with nonstick spray. Add vegetables and cook for 2 minutes, until soft. Pour in eggs, and cook until firm. Sprinkle with cheese. Cook until cheese melts.

SPINACH, ARTICHOKE, AND SUN-DRIED TOMATO FRITTATA

PREP TIME: 20 minutes. **COOKING TIME:** 20 minutes. Serves 6 to 8.

1 tbsp. extra-virgin olive oil	3 tbsp. sun-dried tomatoes, drained and thinly sliced
½ cup sweet onion, finely chopped	
3 cloves garlic, minced	1 tsp. basil
½ cup artichokes, chopped	1 tsp. thyme
1 (10-oz.) bag organic baby spinach	sea salt and freshly cracked pepper to taste
5 large organic eggs	
4 large organic egg whites	4 oz. cracked pepper goat cheese, crumbled
¼ cup fat-free organic milk	

Preheat oven to 400° F. Heat a large, ovenproof skillet over medium heat. Add olive oil and sauté onion and garlic until soft. Add artichokes and spinach. Cook until spinach wilts. Add a little water if needed. In a mixing bowl, whisk together eggs, egg whites, milk, sun-dried tomatoes, basil, and thyme. Season with salt and pepper. Pour into skillet. Use a spatula to lift the spinach and artichokes to allow the eggs to spread underneath. Cook over medium heat until eggs are just set. Sprinkle with goat cheese and place in the oven. Bake for 15 to 20 minutes, until set.

QUINOA BREAKFAST CEREAL

COOKING TIME: 10 minutes. Serves 5.

1 cup organic quinoa	½ tsp. cinnamon
2 cups water	organic plain yogurt
½ cup apples, thinly sliced	fresh berries (optional)
⅓ cup organic raisins	

Rinse quinoa. In a medium saucepan, bring quinoa and water to a boil. Reduce heat and simmer for 5 minutes. Add apples, raisins, and cinnamon. Continue to simmer until water is absorbed (about 10 minutes). Serve with a dollop of yogurt, if desired. Top with fresh berries for an extra treat.

SMOOTHIES

Smoothies are a terrific way to enjoy the wonderful health benefits of green foods.

To increase their nutrient value even more, add a scoop of PEP (polysaccharide Peptide blend) or Super Berry Powder.

These delicious smoothie recipes are courtesy of Judy Brown, the East Coast and Midwest Sales Manager for Green Foods Corporation. Judy holds a Masters Degree in Consumer Economics and has written many articles on food and nutrition. She is the author of *The Natural Lunchbox—Vegetarian Meals for School, Work, and Home,* and *Flax—The Superfood* (see Resources section).

POMEGRANATE BERRY SMOOTHIE

Makes 2 cups.

1 cup organic unsweetened pomegranate juice

½ cup frozen organic blueberries

8 fresh or frozen strawberries

2 teaspoons Green Magma barley grass juice powder

Blend all ingredients until smooth.

ACAI POMEGRANATE SMOOTHIE

Makes 2 servings (1¾ cup).

1 cup pure organic unsweetened pomegranate juice

½ cup (1 packet) pure, organic, unsweetened frozen Acai

8 fresh or frozen strawberries

2 teaspoons Green Magma barley grass juice powder

Blend all ingredients until smooth.

ACAI STRAWBERRY SMOOTHIE

Perricone readers may be surprised to see a recipe with apple juice. However, unsweetened apple juice comes in at 40 on the glycemic index, which makes it an acceptable choice for the smoothie recipe. Just remember, when eating fruit or making smoothies don't drink or eat on an empty stomach. Eat some protein first to prevent a rise in blood sugar.

Makes 2 servings (1¾ cup).

1 cup organic unsweetened apple juice

½ cup (1 packet) pure organic unsweetened frozen Acai

8 fresh or frozen strawberries

2 teaspoons Green Magma barley grass juice powder

Blend all ingredients until smooth.

POMEGRANATE BANANA MAGMA SMOOTHIE

Makes 2 servings (1¾ cup).

½ cup pomegranate juice

½ cup water

2 bananas, peeled and frozen

4 frozen strawberries

2 tsp. Green Magma barley grass juice powder

Blend all ingredients until smooth.

BERRY MAGMA SMOOTHIE

Makes 2 cups.

1 cup water

8 fresh or frozen strawberries

½ cup frozen organic blueberries

2 tsp. organic agave nectar

2 tsp. Green Magma barley grass juice powder

Blend all ingredients until smooth.

Resources

To receive updates on the latest health, beauty, and anti-aging news (and more) featured in *Ageless Face, Ageless Mind* visit www.nvperriconemd.com

Topical Anti-Oxidant, Anti-Aging, Anti-Inflammatory Skin Products, Stimulcell™, Stem-Cell-Messenger Products

Topical Carnosine/Antiglycating Agents, Skin-Brightening Products

N. V. Perricone, M.D., Ltd., 888-823-7837 or www.nvperriconemd.com

N. V. Perricone, M.D., Ltd. Flagship Store, 791 Madison Avenue (at 67th St.), New York, NY

Sephora

Select Neiman Marcus

Nordstrom

Select Bloomingdales

Select Saks

Clyde's on Madison (926 Madison Avenue at 74th St., New York, NY)

Henri Bendel

Light Therapy Mask

Call N. V. Perricone, M.D., Therapeutics, 888-823-7837 for more information.

Electric Muscle Stimulation (EMS) Glove

Call N. V. Perricone, M.D., Therapeutics, 888-823-7837 for more information.

Products for Inflammatory Skin Conditions Including Acne

Skin Clear Nutritional Support System

N. V. Perricone, M.D., Therapeutics, 888-823-7837 or
www.nvperriconemd.com

*N. V. Perricone, M.D., Ltd. Flagship Store, 791 Madison Avenue
(at 67th St.), New York, NY*

Problem Skin Topical Products Outpatient Therapy

N. V. Perricone, M.D., Ltd., 888-823-7837 or http://
www.nvperriconemd.com

*N. V. Perricone, M.D., Ltd. Flagship Store, 791 Madison Avenue
(at 67th St.), New York, NY*

Sephora

Select Neiman Marcus

Nordstrom

Select Bloomingdales

Select Saks

Clyde's on Madison (926 Madison Ave. at 74th St., New York, NY)

Henri Bendel

Sun Protection Nonchemical Sunscreen for Face and Body
Active Tinted Moisturizer with SPF 15

N. V. Perricone, M.D., Therapeutics, 888-823-7837 or
www.nvperriconemd.com

N. V. Perricone, M.D., Ltd. Flagship Store, 791 Madison Avenue
(at 67th St.), New York, NY

Sephora

Select Neiman Marcus

Nordstrom

Select Bloomingdales

Select Saks

Clyde's on Madison (926 Madison Avenue at 74th St., New York, NY)

Henri Bendel

Libido/Energy/Well-Being Enhancers

Neuropeptide/Pheromone Therapeutic Anti-Aging Fragrance
This unique patented formula combines pheromones with a fragrance
rich in therapeutic botanical essences. This results in a therapeutic mood
enhancer and libido booster that also can greatly enhance memory and
mental clarity, lift depression, increase self-confidence, and increase
one's attractiveness to the opposite sex. Additionally, because the limbic
portion of the brain controls autonomous body functions, these fra-
grances can also lower blood pressure; increase blood flow to the brain,
eliminating the confusion that sometimes plagues older people; increase
problem-solving skills; reduce levels of the stress hormones cortisol and
adrenaline, and actually slow the aging process. To learn more about Synergy see *Dr. Perricone's 7 Secrets to Beauty, Health, and Longevity.*

N. V. Perricone, M.D., Ltd., 888-823-7837 or
www.nvperriconemd.com

N. V. Perricone, M.D., Ltd. Flagship Store, 791 Madison Avenue (at 67th St.), New York, NY

Sephora

Select Neiman Marcus

Nordstrom

Select Bloomingdales

Select Saks

Clyde's on Madison (926 Madison Avenue at 74th St., New York, NY)

Henri Bendel

Antiglycating Agents

Benfotiamine
Carnosine
Pyridoxamine
CoQ-10
Glutathione

N. V. Perricone, M.D., Therapeutics, 888-823-7837 or www.nvperriconemd.com

N. V. Perricone, M.D., Ltd. Flagship Store, 791 Madison Avenue (at 67th St.), New York, NY

Glutathione

N. V. Perricone, M.D., Therapeutics, 888-823-7837 or www.nvperriconemd.com

N. V. Perricone, M.D., Ltd. Flagship Store, 791 Madison Avenue (at 67th St.), New York, NY

Total Skin and Body Oral Wrinkle-Reducing Supplements

N. V. Perricone, M.D., Ltd., 888-823-7837 or www.nvperriconemd.com

N. V. Perricone, M.D., Ltd. Flagship Store, 791 Madison Avenue
(at 67th St.), New York, NY

Sephora

Select Neiman Marcus

Nordstrom

Select Bloomingdales

Select Saks

Clyde's on Madison (926 Madison Ave. at 74th St., New York, NY)

Henri Bendel

Weight Management/Blood-Sugar Stabilizers

Weight Management Program Supplements
Chromate® brand of Chromium
Maitake D-Fraction and SX-Fraction Extract
Conjugated Linoleic Acid (CLA)
Coenzyme Q-10
Carnitine and Acetyl-L-Carnitine
Alpha Lipoic Acid
Gamma Linoleic Acid (GLA)
L-Glutamine Powder

N. V. Perricone, M.D., Ltd., 888-823-7837 or
www.nvperriconemd.com

N. V. Perricone, M.D. Ltd. Flagship Store, 791 Madison Avenue
(at 67th St.), New York, NY

High-quality Fish-Oil Capsules

N. V. Perricone, M.D., Ltd., 888-823-7837 or
www.nvperriconemd.com

*N. V. Perricone M.D., Ltd. Flagship Store, 791 Madison Avenue (at 67th St.),
New York, NY*

Vital Choice Seafood, 800-608-4825, www.vitalchoice.com

Optimum Health International, 800-228-1507 www.opthealth.com

Nutritional Supplements/Mitochondrial Rejuvenators

Anti-aging, Anti-inflammatory Supplements
Skin and Total Body Nutritional Supplements, formulated by
N. V. Perricone, M.D., are available from:

N. V. Perricone, M.D., Ltd., 888-823-7837 or
www.nvperriconemd.com

N. V. Perricone M.D., Ltd. Flagship Store, 791 Madison Avenue
(at 67th St.), New York, NY

Sephora

Select Neiman Marcus

Nordstrom

Select Bloomingdales

Select Saks

Clyde's on Madison (926 Madison Ave. at 74th St., New York, NY)

Henri Bendel

Optimum Health International, 800-228-1507 or www.opthealth.com

Life Extension Foundation, 800-544-4440 or www.lef.org

AstaREAL™ Astaxanthin Supplements

N. V. Perricone, M.D., Ltd., 888-823-7837 or
www.nvperriconemd.com

CAN-C Carnosine Eye Drops
IAS Group.(International Aging Systems), www.antiaging-systems.com

Name: International Antiaging Systems
Address: IAS House, PO Box 6, Dept. P, Sark GY9 0SB, Great Britain
Phone (USA) 415-992-5563 (UK) 0208.123.2106
Fax (USA) 415-366-1503 (UK) 0208.181.6106
Email: ias@antiaging-systems.com
Website: www.antiaging-systems.com
Note: Mention Dr. Perricone and get free shipping and handling on your first order.

Pyridoxamine—The Rare Anti-aging B Vitamin
IAS Group www.antiaging-systems.com

Name: International Antiaging Systems
Address: IAS House, PO Box 6, Dept. P, Sark GY9 0SB, Great Britain
Phone (USA) 415-992-5563 (UK) 0208.123.2106
Fax (USA) 415-366-1503 (UK) 0208.181.6106
Email: ias@antiaging-systems.com
Website: www.antiaging-systems.com
Note: Mention Dr. Perricone and get free shipping and handling on your first order.

Pycnogenol
Exclusive North American Distributor, Natural Health Science, Inc., Hoboken NJ. Today, Pycnogenol® is available in more than 600 dietary supplements, multivitamins, cosmeceuticals, and functional foods and beverages worldwide. Pycnogenol® products are available at your local health food store, drugstore, and grocery store, and on the Internet.

For more information, please visit their website at www.pycnogenol.com

Rhodiola—Arctic Root®
Arctic Root is made from a unique extract of Rhodiola rosea (SHR-5) and developed for stress relief, mental clarity, energy, and positive mood support. There is only one Arctic Root, produced after 30 years of research, clinical trials, and safety studies by the Swedish Herbal Institute.

For more information and to order visit www.proactivebio.com

Resveratrol

Enzymatic Therapy
Enzymatic Therapy, Inc., 825 Challenger Drive, Green Bay, WI 54311,
www.enzy.com

Vitacost
NSI Resveratrol—100 mg
NSI Grape Seed Extract with Resveratrol—120 mg
NSI Resveratrol Green Tea, C, Grape Complex
www.vitacost.com

Bullwater Health & Fitness
Pomology Anti-Aging with Resveratrol formula
www.pomology.com/

Country Life
www.country-life.com/

Jarrow Formulas
www.jarrow.com/main.php

Supplements for Bone Health and Cardiovascular Support

Vitamin K2

Vitamin K2/Bone Solutions

Advanced Biosolutions, 888-887-7498 or www.drsinatra.com

Choline-stabilized orthosilicic acid (ch-OSA™), Jarrow Formulas®
BioSil™, available at www.jarrow.com

P 73 Oregano and Related Products

Oil of oregano is an herbal product that has been used since biblical times.
It was widely used in ancient Greece for many medical purposes. Oil of

oregano is a potent antiseptic, meaning that it kills germs. Research proves that it is highly effective for killing a wide range of fungi, yeast, and bacteria, including MRSA and avian bird flu, as well as parasites and viruses.

North American Herb & Spice, 800-243-5242 or www.oreganol.com

Recommended reading:

Natural Cures for Killer Germs and *The Cure is in the Cupboard* by Dr. Cass Ingram (www.amazon.com)

Starch and Sugar Blockers
Phase 2 Starch Blockers

Natrol's Carb Intercept and Slenderlite, available at drugstores, supermarkets, and natural food stores

Contact Carb-Ease to find a distributor near you: www.advocare.com

Recommended Foods

Wild Alaskan salmon/tuna/halibut/sardines; wild organic blueberries; organic dark chocolate; organic herbs and spices; organic teas; salmon sausage and burgers

Vital Choice Seafood. Wild Alaskan salmon has a healthier fatty-acid profile (less saturated fat, higher ratio of omega-3 fatty acids to saturated fats), compared with farmed salmon. Vital Choice Seafood products (salmon, tuna, and halibut) are caught at sea, flash-frozen immediately, packed in dry ice, and delivered via FED EX or UPS at affordable prices. In 2000, wild Alaskan salmon was the first fishery certified as sustainable by the Marine Stewardship Council. www.vitalchoice.com or 800-608-4825.

Acai (Amazonian fruit high in antioxidants)

Acai fruit has more antioxidants than wild blueberries, pomegranate, or red wine; it also contains essential omegas (healthy fats), amino acids, calcium, and fiber.

Super Berry Powder with Acai
A berry powder drink containing high amounts of antioxidants and anti-inflammatories. Both qualities maintain cell health and protection from free radical damage, and provide support to the major organ functions in the body. Contains acai, ranked as the #1 Super Food in Dr. Perricone's book *The Perricone Promise.*

> N. V. Perricone, M.D., Ltd., 888-823-7837, www.nvperriconemd.com

> *N. V. Perricone M.D. Ltd., Flagship Store, 791 Madison Avenue (at 67th St.) New York, New York*

> Sambazon brand Acai beverages can also be found nationwide at Whole Foods Market and Wild Oats stores www.sambazon.com

Avocado
Recipes, health information, the California Avocado Board, www.avocado.org

Beans and Lentils
Westbrae Naturals markets certified organic beans, including rare heirloom varieties, nationwide. Go to www.westbrae.com/products/index.html or call 800-434-4246.

Carbolina Penne Pasta with Phase 2 Starch Blocker
www.molinarimills.com

Coconut Oil
www.spectrumorganics.com

Foods Alive Organic Golden Flax Crackers (grain free)
www.foodsalive.com

Organic Dairy and Cheeses
www.organicvalleycoop.com

Organic Valley is organic and farmer-owned since 1988.

This co-op of more than 1100 farmers produces the finest organic products, including milk, yogurt, and cheese. They are widely available in natural food stores and natural food sections of supermarkets. To find a store near you, visit their website.

Goat and Sheep Dairy Products
Redwood Hill Farms
www.redwoodhills.com

This company's delicious goat milk yogurt and fine artisanal cheeses are naturals for cooking. Try using their goat milk yogurt in almost any recipe that calls for milk, cream, sour cream, or buttermilk. Their cheeses, fresh or aged, soft or crumbly, spreadable or hard, are perfect for any course. Goat cheese, like goat milk, is easier on the human digestive system and lower in calories, cholesterol, and fat than its bovine counterpart. Goat cheese is also rich in calcium, protein, vitamin A, vitamin K, phosphorus, niacin, and thiamine. Their website also has great recipes.

The Coonridge Organic Goat Cheese Dairy
www.coonridge.com

Since 1981 the Coonridge Organic Goat Cheese Dairy has been altering the dynamics of natural cheeses. They offer a choice with superior flavor and full nutrition in reusable packaging. Coonridge proves that wonderful taste and nutritional superiority don't have to come at the expense of the environment, the goat's health, or your health. Besides promoting sustainable, nonchemical, non–factory farmed animal husbandry and cheesemaking, they strive to always live in harmony with the natural world that supports us all.

Feta Cheese
www.malincho.com

Order online or call 866-203-3525. This company has outstanding goat feta cheese from the Balkans that is tremendously flavorful. It also has many other products.

Grating Cheeses from Italy including Pecorino Romano and parmigiano Reggiano
www.formaggio-kitchen.com

From the high-mountain cheeses of Valle d'Aosta through the foggy Piedmont, on to Tuscany and the islands of Sicily and Sardinia, Italy's cheeses offer variety not only in size and shape but also in texture and flavor.

Kefir and Yogurt

Helios Nutrition is a small organic dairy in Sauk Centre, Minnesota that makes several flavors of organic kefir with added FOS (a prebiotic polysaccharide). Locate retail outlets at 888-3 HELIOS or www.heliosnutrition.com/html/where_to_buy.html

Stonyfield Farm yogurt is available at many food markets. See the store locator at www.stonyfield.com/StoreLocator/

Horizon Organic yogurt is available at many food markets. See the store locator at www.horizonorganic.com/findingproducts/index.html

Diamond Organics, Inc. sells organic yogurt direct to consumers at www.diamondorganics.com/dairy.html#straus

Goji Berry

The Tibetan Goji Berry Company

All goji berries supplied worldwide are processed through the office of the Tibetan Goji Berry Company. This single-source supply office works for botanical conservation and to protect against overharvesting of this limited crop of wildcrafted goji berry. Available at 866-328-4654 or www.GojiBerry.com.

100% Grass-Fed Beef
www.eatwild.com/

Eatwild.com is your source for safe, healthy, natural, nutritious grass-fed beef, lamb, goat meat, bison meat, poultry, pork, and dairy products. This site has three goals: to link consumers with reliable suppliers of all-natural, delicious, grass-fed products; to provide comprehensive, accurate information about the benefits of raising animals in pastures; and to provide a marketplace for farmers who raise their livestock in pastures from birth to market, and who actively promote the welfare of their animals and the health of the land.

Neff Family Ranch Offers 100% Grass-fed Beef Grazed in Organic Pastures.
www.nfrnaturalbeef.com

Recommended Reading:

Dr. Perricone's 7 Secrets to Beauty, Health, and Longevity, Nicholas Perricone, M.D., Ballantine Books, New York, 2006. www.amazon.com

The Perricone Weight Loss Diet, Nicholas Perricone, M.D., Ballantine Books, New York, 2005. www.amazon.com

The Perricone Promise, Nicholas Perricone, M.D., Warner Books, 2004.

The Clear Skin Prescription, Nicholas Perricone, M.D., HarperCollins, 2003.

The Perricone Prescription, Nicholas Perricone, M.D., HarperCollins, 2002.

The Wrinkle Cure, Nicholas Perricone, M.D., Warner Books, 2001.

The Natural Weight Loss Pharmacy, Harry Preuss, M.D., MACN, CNS, and Bill Gottlieb, Broadway Books, 2007, www.amazon.com

Maitake Magic, Harry Preuss, M.D., MACN, CNS, and Sensuke Konno, Freedom Press, 2002, www.amazon.com

Pasture Perfect: The Far-Reaching Benefits of Choosing Meat, Eggs, and Dairy Products from Grass-Fed Animals, Jo Robinson, www.eatwild.com

The Omnivore's Dilemma, Michael Pollen. Available at bookstores, www.amazon.com, and www.eatwild.com.

Green Barley Essence: The Ideal Fast Food, Dr. Yoshihide Hagiwara, McGraw-Hill, Hightstown, NJ, 1985.

Green Leaves of Barley: Nature's Miracle Rejuvenator, Dr. Mary Ruth Swope and David A. Darbro, M.D., Swope Enterprises, Lone Star, TX 1996.

Wheat Grass: Nature's Finest Medicine, Steve Meyerowitz, Sproutman Publications, Great Barrington, MA, 1998. www.amazon.com

Note: This book is actually about cereal grasses, not just wheatgrass, and it contains a large section of scientific research on the health benefits of barley grass juice.

Barley Grass Juice: Rejuvenation Elixir and Natural, Healthy Power Drink, Barbara Simonsohn, Lotus Press, Twin Lakes, WI 2001.

Green Foods

Certified organic barley grass, Green Magma powder and supplements. Available at natural food stores, including Whole Foods and Wild Oats. For additional retailers and online retailers visit www.greenfoods.com

Green Tea
For high-quality teas (green, white, and black) with the highest polyphenol content

The Yau Hing Company, 415-395-0868 www.YHTEAS.com

888-ORGANIC (888-674-2642).

Green Tea Extract
The active constituents in green tea are polyphenols, with an antioxidant called epigallocatechin 3 gallate (EGCG) being the most powerful. You can find many products in drug and natural food stores listed as either green tea extract or EGCG. Shogun Imperial Green Tea, the world's most potent green tea, is available in capsule form at local drug and natural foods stores or at www.greenfoods.com. Life Extension has a mega green tea extract available at www.lef.org.

Teavigo Pure, Natural Potent Green Tea Extract
DSM Nutritional Products www.dsm.com

Organic Fruits and Vegetables Delivered to Your Home

Diamond Organics, Inc. sells certified organic berries (in season, May through October) direct to consumers. Go to www.diamondorganics.com or call 888-ORGANIC (888-674-2642).

Organic Markets Nationwide

For fish, poultry, other meats, eggs, fruits, vegetables, barley, oats, buckwheat, beans, lentils, hot peppers, nuts, seeds, extra-virgin olive oil, herbs, spices, spring water, tea (green, white, and black), nutritional supplements, kefir, yogurt, etc.

Whole Foods Market has an outstanding choice of natural and organic foods. Log on to their website to find a store near you, www.wholefoods.com.

Wild Oats is another national chain offering an excellent selection of organic and natural food. To find a store near you visit www.wildoats.com.

Polysaccharide Peptide Food Products (anti-inflammatory and anti-aging)

N. V. Perricone, M. D., Ltd., 888-823-7837 or www.nvperriconemd
.com

N. V. Perricone, M. D., Ltd. Flagship Store, 791 Madison Avenue
(at 67th St.), New York, NY

Pistachio Nuts

California Pistachio nuts www.everybodysnuts.com. Found in supermarkets and grocery stores nationwide.

Pomegranate Juice and Concentrate (Extremely High in Antioxidants)

POM Wonderful at 310-966-5800 or www.pomwonderful.com
Also available at supermarkets and natural food stores.

Pure Spring Water

Poland Spring water, found in supermarkets and grocery stores
nationwide.

Fiji water natural artesian water bottled at its source in the Fijian
islands, available at leading grocery and convenience chains. Fiji
water is also available for home delivery in the continental U.S. at
www.fijiwater.com.

Sea Vegetables

Maine Coast Sea Vegetables, www.seaveg.com

Eden Foods, www.edenfoods.com

Sprouts: Information and Supplies

The International Sprout Growers Association (ISGA) at www .isgasprouts.org is a professional association of sprout growers and companies that supplies products and services to the sprout industry. Visit their website for outstanding information, recipes, and health notes.

Turmeric Extract

New Chapter, Inc. markets the high-potency turmeric extract TurmericForce. www.new-chapter.com or 800-543-7279.

Most natural food stores and grocers also carry fresh turmeric root.

Recipes

www.wildoats
I would like to thank Judy Brown, who is the East Coast and Midwest Sales Manager for Green Foods Corporation, for creating these delicious smoothie recipes. Judy holds a Masters degree in consumer economics. She is also the author of *The Natural Lunchbox—Vegetarian Meals for School, Work and Home*, and *Flax—The Superfood*, published by the Book Publishing Company, 800-695-2241.
Judy has published more than 40 articles on natural foods.

Recommended Cookware and Bakeware

It should come as no surprise that my favorite cookware and bakeware hail from France, one of the countries most famed for superior cuisine. The cookware that you choose is very important to your health as well as to the flavor of your food. Porcelain and enamel cookware will not interact with your food, which is particularly important when you are dealing with acidic foods such as vinegar and lemon. Avoid nonstick cookware and bakeware. Although the recommend items cost a bit more, if properly cared for they will last a lifetime—a wise investment that you only have to make once.

Emile Henry Cookware
www.emilehenry.com.

The Burgundy region of France is the home of Emile Henry cookware. Since 1850 five generations of the Henry family have been handcrafting this famous oven-to-tableware. Since it was first produced, the major benefit of cooking in oven-to-tableware has been its ability to allow gradual, even heat distribution through the food so the fibers soften slowly, without toughening. Available at fine stores such as Williams-Sonoma. For a complete listing of retail and online listings, visit their website.

Le Creuset
Le Creuset is the world's leading manufacturer of enamel cast-iron cookware. Like Emile Henry, Le Creuset is as beautiful as it is functional. All the Le Creuset cookware is made from enamel cast iron, which has been used for cooking utensils since the middle ages. In 1925, the foundry began producing cast iron by hand-casting molten cast iron in sand molds, still the most delicate stage of the production process. Even today, after casting, each mold is destroyed, and the cookware is polished and sanded by hand, then scrutinized for imperfections. Once declared good for enameling, the items are sprayed with two separate coats of enamel and fired after each process at a temperature of 800° C. The enamel then becomes extremely hard and durable, making it almost completely resistant to damage during normal use. Since much of the finishing is done by hand, each Le Creuset Cast Iron cookware piece is completely unique.

Recommended Household Products

Seventh Generation
There is an alternative to toxic cleansers and environmentally unfriendly paper and plastic. I recommend Seventh Generation, which offers a complete line of nontoxic household products. All their products are designed to work as well as their traditional counterparts, but use renewable, non-

toxic, phosphate-free, and biodegradable ingredients, and are never tested on animals. They are as gentle on the planet as they are on people, and they don't create fumes or leave residues that may affect the health of your family or pets. Seventh Generation products are widely available nationwide. To learn more and find a retailer or online retailer, visit www.seventhgeneration.com.

Health Education Information

These websites offer interesting information on the topics of nutrition, natural healing, food, and holistic health.

IAS Group is an outstanding source for anti-aging medicine, nutrition, and information.

Name: International Antiaging Systems
Address: IAS House, PO Box 6, Dept. P, Sark GY9 0SB, Great Britain
Phone (USA) 415-992-5563 (UK) 0208.123.2106
Fax (USA) 415-366-1503 (UK) 0208.181.6106
E-mail: ias@antiaging-systems.com
Website: www.antiaging-systems.com
Note: Mention Dr. Perricone and get free shipping and handling on your first order.

For up-to-the minute scientific news and information on food and nutritional supplements, including the latest on the weight-loss benefits of sesame seed, visit www.lef.org.

The European Food Information Council (EUFIC) is a nonprofit organization that provides science-based information on food and food-related topics to the media, health and nutrition professionals, educators, and opinion leaders. www.eufic.org

For information on the glycemic index, visit www.glycemicindex.com.

For excellent information on general health and nutrition, including different types of meat and sugars, visit www.mercola.com.

For information on the cancer-preventing phytonutrients found in fruits and vegetables, visit the American Institute for Cancer Research at www.aicr.org.

For outstanding information on the benefits and various types of exercise, including detailed information with drawings, visit the following websites: the President's Council on Physical Fitness (PCPFS), www.fitness.gov and the National Institute of Aging, www.niapublications.org.

Health Benefits of Olive Oil

www.iooc.com

Nonglycemic Sweeteners

To learn more about the pros and cons of all available sweeteners, both natural and chemical, visit www.holisticmed.com/sweet.

For information on stevia, visit www.stevia.net.

For information on ZSweet natural sugar substitute, visit www.eridex.com.

For comprehensive information on soy foods, visit www.soyfoods.com.

To learn about seafood safety, visit the Union of Concerned Scientists, www.ucsusa.org; the Federal Food and Drug Administration (FDA) food safety website, www.cfsan.fda.gov/~frf/sea-mehg.html; and the Environmental Protection Agency (EPA), www.epa.gov/ost/fish, www.epa.gov/mercury, or www.vitalchoice.com.

Index

NICHOLAS PERRICONE, M.D., is the #1 *New York Times* bestselling author whose books include *Dr. Perricone's 7 Secrets to Beauty, Health, and Longevity, The Perricone Weight-Loss Diet, The Wrinkle Cure, The Perricone Prescription,* and *The Perricone Promise.* He is a board certified dermatologist, award-winning inventor, research scientist, and internationally renowned anti-aging expert. He is the focus of a series of award-winning PBS specials, and a popular guest on *The Oprah Winfrey Show, Today, 20/20, Good Morning America,* and *Larry King Live,* among other programs. He is currently adjunct professor of medicine at Michigan State University's College of Human Medicine. Visit the author's website at www.nvperriconemd.com.

ABOUT THE TYPE

The text of this book was set in Filosofia. It was designed in 1996 by Zuzana Licko, who created it for digital type-setting as an interpretation of the sixteenth-century typeface Bodoni. Filosofia, an example of Licko's un-usual font designs, has classical proportions with a strong feeling, softened by rounded droplike serifs. She has designed many typefaces and is the cofounder of *Emigre* magazine, where many of them first appeared. Born in Bratislava, Czechoslovakia, Licko came to the United States in 1968. She studied graphic communi-cations at the University of California at Berkeley, graduating in 1984.